"What happens when a nature writer turns their attention to the most unnerving of all landscapes – those that exist in our bodies and minds? Nic Wilson has done just that, exploring internal thickets of tangled nature and nurture, wild gardens where the composted past feeds the present, marshes of intermingled memory and meaning. The result is a book of great courage, curiosity, discovery and connection."
Amy-Jane Beer, author of *The Flow*

"Both ordinary and profound, *Land Beneath the Waves* charts a process most of us never manage: to give a true account of ourselves. It's also an illuminating testimony of chronic illness, one that fellow sufferers will recognise and the rest of us can only be enlarged by."
Melissa Harrison, novelist, nature writer and children's author

"A beautiful, moving memoir highlighting the amazing relationships humans have with the natural world, and what they mean for us."
Kate Bradbury, author, journalist and TV presenter

"A deeply honest, forensically detailed account of a life blighted by ill-health, yet redeemed by a profound connection with nature – a delight to read."
Stephen Moss, author and naturalist

"*Land Beneath the Waves* is a tender portrait of how a family grows in tandem with the natural world. The body, here, is re-storied: it becomes both objects of contemplation in Nic Wilson's quest to make sense of chronic illness across generations, and the stage for vital, lively connection with plants, water, land, and place. It is hopeful, vibrant, and alive."
Jessica J. Lee, author and environmental historian

"A moving, honest and compassionate story of illness, and the beauty and succour to be found in the natural world. Nic reveals the complexity of our relationships with wildlife and landscapes, which does not simply offer a cure but can help us meet the challenges of chronic ill health."
Patrick Barkham, author of *Wild Child*

"When our health fails, nature seems harsh, yet in *Land Beneath the Waves* Nic Wilson offers a tender love song to both the body and the wild world, even when – especially when – both are under threat. Exploring the complex territories of debilitating illness, motherhood and finding healing in nature, her writing reclaims the great outdoors for those who so often are shut in. Hopeful and brave."
Merryn Glover, author of *Of Stone and Sky*

"This one's different. It's not another book about the soothing power of the wild (view them with suspicion) but a taut, unself-pitying inquiry into the nature of nature, the nature of suffering, the caprice of memory and the slipperiness of identity: a sort of theodicy that mentions nightingales but not God. Nothing in the real, living world is incidental, and because the book is a real, living thing, nothing here is incidental either. It's a tightly woven ecosystem of woods, anxiety, hedges and hope. It will endure long after more emollient books have been pulped."

Charles Foster, author of *Cry of the Wild*

"A powerful record of the way joy in the natural world may counterbalance intergenerational illness and systemic failures. Through reconciling long-buried childhood experiences and accepting the complex reality of her own body, Nic Wilson offers a vital retort to 'the myth that worthwhile encounters with the natural world only happen to wild people in wild places'. An important and necessary addition to writing about nature and illness."

Polly Atkins, author of *Some of Us Just Fall*

"A brave and beautifully written memoir of a life lived close to nature, despite the significant challenges imposed by chronic illness and pain. In *Land Beneath the Waves* Nic Wilson courageously explores the fragmented memories of her past, to better understand her relationships with herself, her family, and the natural world; a journey both deeply moving and full of hope. I loved this book."

Brigit Strawbridge Howard, author of *Dancing with Bees*

"I loved *Land Beneath the Waves*. An honest and touching memoir, beautifully observed and written, and a wonderful advertisement for the importance of connection with the natural world."
Lev Parikian, writer and conductor

"The natural world beats to its own rhythm, and when we tune in, we change state to become part of something much bigger than ourselves. When facing daily pain, both mental and physical, that can be a godsend. In *Land Beneath the Waves*, Nic Wilson demonstrates with gritty realism and deep feeling just how important nature is, no matter what our state of health. A moving book with depth and perception, and laced through with hope. Nature as friend, comforter and counsellor."
Mary Colwell, environmentalist author and producer

"A brutally honest story that demonstrates why nature keeps us afloat. Nic Wilson is one of the most exciting emerging nature writers; her debut is an unstoppable tide, washing over the reader with pain but always with joy and kindness."
Jack Wallington, author and landscape and garden designer

"An incredible journey, beautifully written, of nature's transformative powers."
Benedict Macdonald, author of *Rebirding*

"With Nic Wilson's memory fragmented, her story is one that illustrates how our deep connection with the world around us is innate and how, irrespective of memory, it has the power to shape who we are. A heartfelt, honest memoir, lovingly told, that will invite you to value the nature on your doorstep."
Hannah Bourne-Taylor, author of *Fledging*

"Touching and beautiful. A courageous reflection on a life spent managing long-term illness and an unreliable body, and the remarkable ways that nature can hold a family together."
Ben Hoare, writer and editor

"I was captivated and deeply moved by this wonderful piece of writing – a balm indeed."
Robin Ince, author and broadcaster

"Nic Wilson guides us time-slipping through her world, guided by botany, birdsong and ancient geology. A journey through overlooked snickets, the edgelands of chronic pain and anxiety and, ultimately, to finding belonging in the margins."
Doreen Cunningham, author of *Soundings*

"A vivid account of intergenerational trauma and how being attuned to nature can help you get through."
Sally Huband, writer and naturalist

Land
Beneath
the
Waves

An Hachette UK Company
www.hachette.co.uk

Summersdale Publishers
Part of Octopus Publishing Group Limited
Carmelite House
50 Victoria Embankment
LONDON
EC4Y 0DZ
UK

www.summersdale.com

The authorized representative in the EEA is Hachette Ireland, 8 Castlecourt Centre, Dublin 15, D15 XTP3, Ireland (email: info@hbgi.ie)

Printed and bound by Clays Ltd, Suffolk, NR35 1ED

ISBN: 978-1-83799-622-3
eISBN: 978-1-83799-623-0

This FSC® label means that materials and other controlled sources used for the product have been responsibly sourced

MIX
Paper | Supporting responsible forestry
FSC
www.fsc.org
FSC® C104740

Substantial discounts on bulk quantities of Summersdale books are available to corporations, professional associations and other organisations. For details contact general enquiries: telephone: +44 (0) 1243 771107 or email: enquiries@summersdale.com.

Land
Beneath
the
Waves

How the natural
world helped one woman
navigate chronic illness,
self-acceptance
and belonging

Nic Wilson

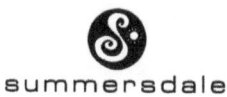

summersdale

Author's Note

I've told my story as honestly as I can based on what I remember. I'm extremely grateful that friends and family have been willing to share their recollections with me during the process of writing. I also used many documents including diaries, journals, scrapbooks, school reports, medical records, stories and poetry I wrote as a child, family photographs and hundreds of letters. On occasion, identifying details have been changed to protect people's privacy.

For my bairns, with all my love

Contents

Bombweed   **19**

Moths at Midnight   **31**

Watcher in the Shadows   **65**

The Wood Between the Worlds   **91**

The Road Less Travelled   **107**

Flatlands   **135**

Grounded   **155**

The BFG   **175**

Snickets   **199**

The Nightingale's Tale   **223**

Inundation   **245**

Chalkbones   **269**

Return to Sea   **295**

References   **301**

Helpful Websites   **307**

Acknowledgements   **309**

About the Author   **313**

Contents

There's rosemary, that's for remembrance; pray, love, remember.

William Shakespeare, *Hamlet*

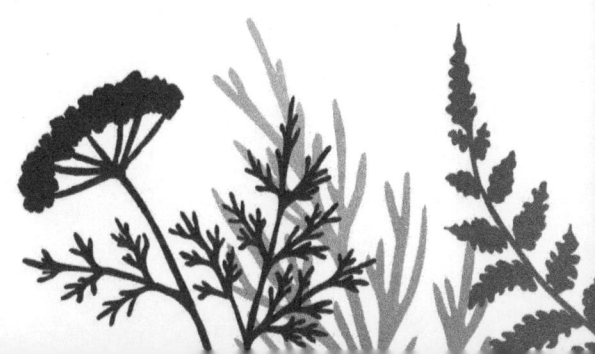

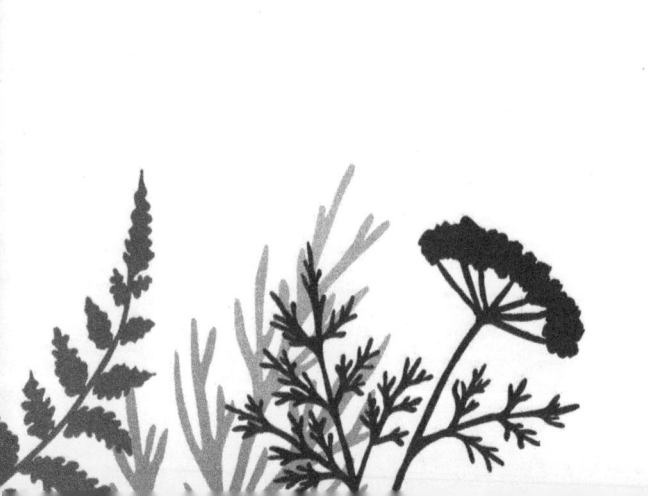

Bombweed

I am not a memoirist. I may as well lay my cards on the table. They make a nine by five grid: one card for every year of my life. Starting at the very beginning, I turn card after card (feel the expectation, the watching eyes, the silence). Draw a line of blanks, a sequence of absence. The negative space is overwhelming. My life is viscous; more often than not it seals itself behind me. Other people offer me their memories, but it feels like make-believe. Fragments of an ordinary life. Perhaps it is mine, perhaps not.

They tell me I lived in a suburban semi set back from the B4114.
They tell me I went to a Catholic primary school.
They tell me I was good at tap and ballet.
They tell me I was happy.

All I remember is the bombweed.

Perhaps it's unsurprising that rosebay willowherb is the only survivor around the edges of my amnesic crater given the plant's infamous reputation for colonising bombsites in the Second World War. Looking back through the smoke, I can see the curling puff of windborne seeds above a thicket of vegetation, the rigid, serried stems, those red-tinged leaves. Bombweed memories so dense they colonise my childhood garden with their rhizomatous roots; they undercut the apple trees, supplant my dad's veg patch, even infiltrate the house, drifting as seed-memories through each room, filling the gaps with a lick of pink flowers.

Seven blank cards in a row. Turning a bright, slow pink.

Mum tells me about a family holiday near Clovelly in Devon. She brings out old photos of me riding a donkey. I try to remember the cottage we stayed in, try to visualise walking down the steep main street to the beach and building castles in the sand with my brother, but it has all gone. Only the smell of Shasta daisies lingers round the cottage door, a pervasive odour of sweaty feet that gripped me by the throat that week and refused to let go.

Even after I've turned those seven blank cards – the childhood years swallowed by my subconscious – my later recollections are still hazy. My husband reminds me of our walks in Provence: the gorges, the metal walkways, the water. I've lost sight of the vistas, but something persists underfoot in the crush of garrigue scrub: a warm, resinous rising of thyme, rosemary, sage. And there was that visit to the Isles of Scilly, he recalls. We took a walk along the cliffs and explored some of the islands by boat. I search for these memories in vain, but I do remember the tall fuchsia hedges lining the narrow roads, my astonishment at their overt floriferousness, like a jeweller's counter of scarlet and purple drop earrings stretching across St Mary's Island. Shake me and the past is erased, we joke. Etch A Sketch me. But not the plants. I remember their scents and flowers, their colours and companionship. I cherish our shared history; it returns to me a little of my forgotten past.

Birdsong evokes memories too. I sat in the garden one sunny May afternoon, a few years ago, with a light wind blowing, listening to distant children playing, an ice cream van sliding up and down its scales and the collared doves calling. Closing my eyes, I was back in Coventry in the 1980s, looking out of the bedroom window in Grandma's small semi-detached house in Tile Hill. The summer stretched before me in its warm laziness and the narrow garden was filled with deckchairs and nattering relatives. The tall conifers at the end of the lawn created an impenetrable wall within whose secure boundaries my memories played out. I remember Grandma's garden for its unforgiving concrete paving slabs, an echoing garage full of cold smells, and the honesty seed heads, each a translucent coin, chocolate-coloured seeds within. When the collared doves lulled me into a trance, I awoke in the little front bedroom and traced the leaves on the wallpaper with my eyes, each with the same toothed edges and green veins scored across the raised leaf blade.

John Lewis-Stempel writes in *Meadowland* that 'birds have a Proustian capacity for making remembrance'. So collared doves pull me to awakenings in that soft-leaved room in Coventry with the summer garden beneath. When herring gulls descant above the slap of the sea, I'm in Granny and Grandpa's loft bedroom in Conwy, watching from beneath a mountain of woollen blankets as birds circle outside the dormer window. These sights, scents and sounds are nature's treasures, ready to enhance the present with layers of wild remembrance. Even the most elusive cue can provoke ripples of recollections, adding emotional depth to a blackbird's song or a flash of buttercups. The memories are papery and thin, and like honesty seed heads some will blow away, but I can see through the layers to the kernels within. When I watch my children gathering cow parsley posies on the way to school or running their hands through the dead-nettle leaves, thrilled, waiting for the half-anticipated sting that never comes, I hope they're collecting their own wild memories for the future.

I don't know how or when I lost the first seven and a half years of my life. And I don't need to know.

This is a lie, of course, but one I've told myself so often it feels like a truth. Those seven blank cards secretly trouble me. My memory has always been poor, but those early years feel different, as if something vital has been erased and I've forgotten what it is. My childhood is hollow and confusing; thinking about it makes my head ache. I prefer to write about the lives of birds, trees and poets, or the histories of landscapes and their inhabitants. Narratives that stay put and don't try to change me. I'm fascinated by the natural history of my local area, and the more I learn about the streets, gardens and marginal spaces around me – even the sky outside my window, which is sometimes all I can see for days on end – the more these ordinary settings reveal to me the extraordinary power of the local, the familiar, the quotidian. At times it feels like the past is seeping into the present-day landscape: squeezing through pavement cracks, sprouting in the verges, sending up vegetative reminders on the peripheries of modernised gardens, submerging our 'now' beneath layers of *natural* history. As I walk down my road, the turned earth of the old field strips and noise of the chalk quarry sometimes seem more real than the houses and traffic that surround me. It's not that I don't belong in the present, more that I sense an affinity with the past and begin to see its role in shaping the land. The future, however, remains obscure. I can't sense it in the landscape and perhaps that's just as well.

I've been making notes on the area around my house for several years now – writing about my walks, visiting the North Hertfordshire Museum and Herbarium, researching naturalists who lived here, reading natural history journals and field notebooks from centuries past, all with the intention of writing a book on wildlife and landscape. But my words fall flat on the page. Though I give a voice to the natural history of the nearby wild, I remain tight-lipped about my own history. I want to argue that it is vital to unearth the past in order to understand how we have arrived in the present. I want to ask how, without an awareness of local landscape history, without some sense of what once existed – those plants, animals, habitats that we have disregarded, forgotten and destroyed – we can ever truly assess the legacy we're leaving for future generations. I want to explore what the land means to me and why. And what it could, or possibly should, mean to every one of us.

But the writing recoils, striking back with personal questions. "Why so much walking into the past and your imagination?" it demands. "What are you trying to escape? Without knowledge of *your* lost years – all those things *you've* ignored and forgotten for so long – how can you understand the legacy *you* are leaving for future generations?"

I cannot sidestep the questions – they interrogate me from the top of every blank page. Why am I so afraid to write about myself? I know the answer really, even if I pretend not to. Before I can write honestly about the wildlife and the local landscape, I must enter my own past. I must face up to my relationship with chronic illness and explore parts of my childhood that I've excised from my memory. And I need to go further back to explore my mother's story and the impact her illness had on me and the family. But these are experiences and feelings I'd far rather leave behind, so I dither in the margins and my writing stagnates. Signing up for this particular expedition seems too high a price to pay for writing a book.

I wonder if I could simply mention my health in passing, noting the way it affects my relationships and confidence, and then move on; but every narrative path leads back to my childhood. I try to follow them dispassionately, as any objective researcher would, but it's no good. I'm a little kid again and I'm falling apart. The speed of my unravelling takes me completely by surprise. The day I embark upon the journey I've been avoiding for months, my journal reads:

Can open; worms everywhere.

I follow the advice of a friend and contact a counsellor. Without the narrative driving me forwards, I fear I'll never find the courage to talk to someone. I don't believe I deserve counselling for my own sake, but I know I'm going to need help if I'm to tell this story.

I begin by tracing my love of the natural world back to my early childhood in Nuneaton. Though I have no memories of our garden, I do have photographs and a letter from my grandma to six-year-old me, mentioning the 'little patch of ground' in which I encountered, first-hand, the magic of plants. I'd imagine my dad was somewhere nearby, perhaps showing me how to mark out my bed or sow my first seeds. Were my parents hoping I'd inherit the green fingers of my forebears? We have gardeners on both sides of the family reaching back for generations. Dad recalls his father's enthusiasm for summer bedding plants and greenhouse tomatoes. He can still remember the smell of fertilisers stored in his father's garage: hoof and horn, superphosphate, sulphate of potash, nitrate of soda, Tonks's rose formula and chalk, all listed in my grandfather's *Fred Streeter Gardeners' Record Book* of 1970 in notes he took the year before he died. My dad attributes his horticultural exploits to his father's love of gardening all those years ago that was then passed down to me, from a grandfather who died four years before I was born.

In my first garden in Nuneaton, I learned early on that wildlife was as important as the crops. Perhaps more so. Photographs show me as a cheerful toddler in red wellingtons playing with sticks and mud, pushing an absurdly big wheelbarrow, sitting in a buggy in a shiny yellow anorak, my face entirely obscured by heavy black binoculars. As I peer at my smaller self down the wrong end of the binoculars, I wonder what the younger me was seeing at that moment. Could I make out the blurry image of my dad to my right, distorted, monstrous, looking back at me through his Praktica L camera? He would have removed the Vivitar 200mm telephoto lens so he could photograph me rather than a bird, but we were still separated by a series of ocular lenses, symbols of this observation of an observation.

I'm holding the binoculars skew-whiff with my chubby two-year-old hands, no doubt mimicking the adults with no clue what I'm doing. I wonder if the photograph was staged for the family album, but I don't think it matters if it was. Only a few years later I'd be using the same binoculars to observe birds in the garden, Dad's reassuring hands clasping mine to steady the image, a shared closeness I felt from the other side this morning as I placed my hands over my son's so he could watch redwings feeding in the cotoneaster.

Staged or not, I love the way the image makes physical my childhood interest in birds. I often write facing those binoculars, the photograph pinned to my noticeboard along with others of me between the ages of two and eight – in the vegetable beds; on Conwy Mountain with Granny's rucksack and a walking stick as tall as my head; embraced by a snug life jacket on Grandpa's boat. These are my talismans against the negative spaces in my memory. I did exist back then. The images are physical proof of my childhood.

Though I rely on photographs and other people's recollections up to the age of seven and a half when we moved from Warwickshire to Cheshire, I still have the rosebay willowherb memories from that first garden. It wasn't until recently that Dad told me this vigorous perennial grew in an uncultivated area at the bottom of our veg plot. Willowherb and other wildflowers thrived there, providing shelter and food for birds, small mammals and invertebrates like moth larvae, including elephant hawk-moth and setaceous Hebrew character, two species that regularly appear on Dad's wildlife lists from the 1970s.

In the summer of 1977, Dad taught himself bricklaying. He ordered a set of precast concrete blocks, 2,000 bricks, 17 tons of scalpings and built a garage next to the house. Photographs from before he began construction show Mum, heavily pregnant with my brother, wielding a spade on top of a huge pile of hardcore. When the garage turned out to be almost too small to fit the car inside (due in Dad's words to a "geometrical misunderstanding"), he transformed the redundant space into a natural history lab filled with bird and mammal skulls, dissected owl pellets, and moths at every stage of life – tiny eggs stuck to leaves, hanging pupae and newly hatched adults ready to be released.

Within a couple of months, Dad had embarked upon a lifelong obsession with lepidoptera that has recently developed a perilous coda. In an idle moment at Birdfair a couple of years ago, I watched with horror as his resolve faltered when faced with a multicoloured array of specialist identification guides. Before I could stop him, he'd bought the *Field Guide to the Micro-moths of Great Britain and Ireland*. I knew there'd be trouble. He'd agreed with Mum long before that micro-moths were a compulsion too far. Not only are there around 1,600 species of micro-moth in the UK, many with a wingspan of less than 20 millimetres, but for a definitive identification it is often necessary to examine the dissected genitalia. Life was too short to peel mushrooms or study micro-moths, Mum reasoned.

But back in 1978 when I was only three, my mum's health was at its lowest ebb and the moth trap was still a shiny new purchase. Dad was enchanted by the moths he discovered upon emptying the trap each morning. Occasionally, he would find eggs laid by gravid females on the underside of the egg boxes placed in the trap to provide shelter. Once he'd begun rearing moths and studying the different instars, or stages of development, there was no going back. Puss moth caterpillars were his favourite. He emails me some of the pictures he took with his Praktica L camera and talks me through them on the phone, the excitement from 40 years ago still evident in his voice:

The puss moth has the most phenomenal caterpillar – a large lime-green larva with a dark brown saddle over the middle and a hump on its back. It's got a red-and-yellow rim around the head, and there are white spiracles, part of the respiratory system, ringed in black along the caterpillar's abdomen. It rears its forked black-and-red tail when threatened and produces a red filament from inside each tail twin that it waves menacingly at you.

I study the caterpillar in the photograph. It is, indeed, a marvel. Dad's second image shows the puss moth at the adult stage, which gives the species its common name. It is clothed in soft ermine with creamy white and black swirls that remind me of the patterns on top of a latte. With its feathered antennae, fluffy face and black-and-white striped legs, it is the embodiment of cuteness in a moth-kitten.

When Dad took me into the garage to see these beauties – the fantastical caterpillar and its fuzzy future – how could I not have shared his fascination? As I watched the puss moth larvae chew willow and poplar bark, combining it with silk to weave tough cocoons from which they would emerge as adult moths in spring, was I ensnared in the warp and weft of their magical lives? Whatever my feelings as a three-year-old, these tiny creatures held the key to my future happiness, because moths saved my parents' marriage.

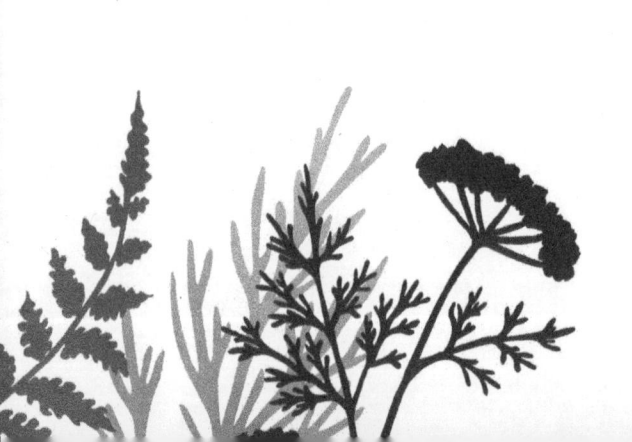

Moths at Midnight

At the end of the first and only consultation, the psychiatrist passed judgement.

"No way can you look after these children," he said to the man who bathed and fed me, who sang 'Down at the Station' to lull me to sleep, who swung me round and round above his head, faster and faster, holding me aloft with his smile. Me and my baby brother.

"They'll have to go into care," the psychiatrist said. "And you" – he turned to my mum – "need to be admitted to a psychiatric unit."

And so the investigation into Mum's illness that had begun three years earlier with the health visitors telling her it was all in her head culminated in the proposed dissolution of my family.

As a child, Mum was no stranger to ill health. She grew up on a council estate in Urmston, 5 miles south-west of Manchester, a second child with a brother five years her senior. Her mother, my granny, couldn't breastfeed, so Mum was given watered-down evaporated milk. Concerned that she was not thriving, the family doctor sent her to the Royal Manchester Children's Hospital, where she was diagnosed with incipient rickets and put on a special formula. After Mum was weaned, Granny would visit the market once a week to buy fresh oranges. It was still three years before rationing ended, so they were expensive and in short supply, but Mum needed the vitamin C. She didn't learn to walk until she was nearly two.

A series of bad throat infections led to the removal of her tonsils when she was just four. Then one afternoon at the age of ten, she tripped over in the school playground and smacked her head on a concrete pillar. She remembers a teacher walking her round the school hall, urging her to stay awake, but after a couple of circuits she passed out. She was unconscious for nearly four hours. I can't help but imagine the scene today if my daughter lost consciousness for that length of time at school: the 999 call, her inert body guided into the recovery position, her classmates ushered away from the windows as she is stretchered into the waiting ambulance. Then the call every parent dreads. The anxious wait in A & E, our shaky relief when she finally comes round. Hospital tests. Her eventual discharge. Compulsive web-searching for warning signs over the coming days. Even as a hypothetical scenario, it gives me the shudders.

Things were somewhat different in 1960. The headmaster drove Mum home in his car and carried her, still unconscious, up to bed. By the time the doctor arrived at 7 p.m., she had come round. When asked how many fingers he was holding up and what time it was, Mum burst into tears. It was Monday evening and she'd missed her piano lesson. She had no tests or follow-up appointments, and remembers nursing an appalling headache that week, as if an orange were being flung backwards and forwards inside her skull.

"Keep her off school for a week," the doctor told her mother. "And make sure she stays quiet for the next twelve months." He wasn't to know it, but his words were prophetic. His advice laid out the pattern of Mum's life for the next 60 years.

After the accident, Mum's energy levels became more erratic. Her blood sugar levels swung from hyper to hypo, and she began to struggle with periods of anxiety and depression. She passed her eleven-plus exam and started at Urmston Grammar School for Girls. Academic success came easily, but in the school holidays she'd retreat to bed to read and recharge her batteries. With no awareness or understanding of energy-limiting illnesses at the time, adults offered little compassion. She always felt under pressure to conceal her exhaustion and act like other children.

During her first year in the sixth form, Mum was offered the chance to go on a school trip around Europe. Led by their physics master, the party camped through Belgium, Germany, Austria, Switzerland and France. None of the girls had ever been abroad before. One hot and humid August night in the Austrian mountains there was a terrible storm. It was the first time Mum had ever experienced simultaneous thunder and lightning. Emerging from their sodden tent in alarm, the girls ran into their teacher in his underpants with his wife and two young daughters; he was on his way to take everyone to safety. He evacuated the group to a farmer's barn where they huddled up in the straw and tried to sleep.

A few days later, Mum found what she thought was an insect bite on her leg haloed by an angry rash – the classic bullseye ring of Lyme disease. Even though symptoms of the disease were first recorded in Europe in the 1880s, it wasn't until the early 1980s that the bacterium that causes Lyme disease was identified, so there was no understanding of the illness or its link to long-term fatigue, and no diagnosis. On her return to England, she was off school for six weeks having come down with yet another infection.

In 1968, she passed her A levels and moved to Birmingham to study law, the first woman in my family to go to university. She managed two terms, but came down with appendicitis in the summer. After a successful appendicectomy, she was discharged from hospital, but within a few days she experienced more unexplained symptoms and was readmitted for further tests. When they all came back negative, the ward sister diagnosed her as a malingerer and told her to get out.

Then, at the beginning of her second year, Mum moved into new digs and met a quiet engineering student with an endearing smile and a wicked sense of humour. Dad and three of his mates had just rented the ground floor of a student house in Edgbaston, on the south-west side of Birmingham. This attractive suburb, developed in the nineteenth century for some of the city's wealthiest industrialists, boasted tree-lined streets with grand neoclassical houses. Dad lived on one of Edgbaston's rougher sides, just down the road from some of the most imposing Victorian residencies, on a back street in the red-light district. Opposite his digs, a Brook Advisory Centre rubbed shoulders with one of the area's many brothels. Punters' cars lined the road, new arrivals always ready to fill any empty parking spaces. Dad got used to the comings and goings, unsought glimpses into other people's private lives. Every week, he'd noticed, a Mini would pull up outside. The driver would get out and disappear inside the brothel, leaving an elderly woman (his mother? Dad wondered) in the passenger seat. Precisely half an hour later, he'd reappear and drive her away. God only knows what the old lady was thinking as she waited in the Mini for him to return. Perhaps he told her he was visiting the dentist for his weekly oral examination.

When four lasses moved into the upstairs rooms, Dad reckoned things might be looking up. His first sight of Mum was of her backside disappearing up the stairs. He recounts this moment with a certain relish, but when I ask him how the first face-to-face meeting went, he is less effusive. "Must have been positive," he surmises, "after all, I asked her out." For their first date, he borrowed a friend's leather jacket so he'd look cool. They went to a party, danced, drank vodka. Back in the house that evening, even though she'd only had a couple of shots, Mum began to feel ill. She threw up all over Dad and the borrowed leather jacket, then passed out. Dad couldn't rouse her. He ran to the phone box down the road to ring for an ambulance. He still remembers the first question the paramedics asked him when they arrived. "I've no idea whether or not she's pregnant," he answered, unnerved. "This is the first time I've been out with her!"

Hospital tests revealed nothing and Mum was discharged again, left to struggle through the rest of the academic year without medical or pastoral support. By the time of her second-year exams, her exhaustion, brain fog and physical weakness meant she was barely able to read or write. Then, at the beginning of her final year, with exam retakes looming, she found herself in the university medical centre awaiting yet more tests. Physically exhausted, unable to think clearly and struggling with depression, she decided enough was enough. She dropped out of university and went to live with Dad and his family. Though she spent a lot of time in bed over the next few weeks, there were short walks on the good days around Limbrick Wood and Coombe Abbey on the outskirts of Coventry. One winter's afternoon, while wandering through a grassy clearing in woodland in Coombe Abbey, Mum and Dad caught a flash of yellow as a large bird took off from the ground and disappeared into the trees. Their first thought was "Golden oriole!" But Dad knew any bird on the ground in the winter wouldn't be an oriole, as it was a rare late-spring visitor. In fact, they'd seen a retreating green woodpecker, which, despite its name, is surprisingly yellow when it reveals its rump in flight. From that moment on, every green woodpecker was a golden oriole – a joking reminder of that first hopeful mistake.

Six months later, after spending time living together, sharing talks, walks and laughter and getting to know each other better through the good times and bad, my parents married and moved into a rented flat in Coventry.

When Dad told Mum he had no hobbies after they'd been together a few months, she pointed out his interest in birds. He was bemused at first. Surely, that was just part of everyday life? But she persuaded him to buy a pair of binoculars and over the next few years this childhood fascination, fostered by *The Observer's Book of British Birds* and days roaming the woods and fields around his rented house in Coventry's Tile Hill, developed into what would become a lifelong passion for nature.

Dad needs quite a bit of persuasion to delve into his early memories. I've inherited my atrocious recollection for family matters from him, our years threaded together instead by natural encounters like bryony berries strung along a hedge. He starts by unearthing a few tales, beginning with his attempt to rear a young starling that had fallen out of its nest under the eaves onto Grandma's back while she was collecting coal from the coal shed. After its narrow escape, Dad kept the starling in the garage, excited by this unexpected opportunity to rear a baby bird. Unfortunately, his plans were thwarted when he went in one morning to find the hapless nestling had strangled itself, having caught its neck between the spokes of his bicycle wheel. His older sister Pauline wrapped the dead starling in a piece of cloth, put it in a shoebox and buried it in the garden. A few days later, wondering if it had gone to heaven yet, she enlisted the help of her friend Barbara to dig up the unfortunate bird. Needless to say, its mortal remains hadn't made it through the pearly gates and both girls got into trouble for their irreverent curiosity.

Dad's other attempts to rear wild animals were equally unsuccessful. Like the time he came across a snake on a Sunday family outing to Lickey Hills, a country park south-west of Birmingham. The poor thing was going about its business in some bracken on the heath when eight-year-old Dad spotted it, scooped it up and took it home. He tells me he tried to feed it on minced beef. Appropriate food, he thought, for such an impressive beast. Turns out he'd caught an elephant hawk-moth caterpillar.

We laugh at his rookie mistake, but he's not the only one to imagine the 8-centimetre larva to be a snake or worse. Nearly every summer the papers seem to run with sensationalist headlines about people who disturb elephant hawk-moth caterpillars, causing them to swell their heads to reveal their large black 'eye' markings, their 'tails' raised as if to strike. Only recently, a couple in Cheshire were advised to call an exorcist after finding one of these magnificent creatures in their garden – a discovery that would make my or my children's day. They're still one of Dad's favourite caterpillars, even though he's not reared them for a few years now, at least not on minced beef. But he's taught his grandchildren to identify the ponderous larvae as they lumber across the lawn in late summer on their way to pupate in the leaf litter.

"What's this?" I ask my daughter, showing her my social media avatar – a muppet-like head with black eye spots, golden eyebrows and a somewhat quizzical expression on its tilted face.

"Elephant hawk-moth caterpillar," she replies without hesitation. Then gives me that look that only your children can. *I'm intrigued by your quirky interests,* her expression says, *but I think you're so weird.*

When I ask Dad what he got up to with his mates in the local fields and hedgerows, he looks sheepish for a moment, like a lad caught with his fingers in the sweetie jar. "Just playing out," he says, "searching the scrub and climbing trees to find bird's nests, at a time when collecting eggs was a normal childhood pastime." Once he clambered up a Scots pine to reach a carrion crow's nest. Getting to his prize was pretty hairy, the thin branches snapping under his hands and feet as he shimmied up the trunk.

Sometimes he'd walk the 3 miles to nearby Berkswell village along the country lanes, birdnesting as he went. He doesn't recall his first day at school, his favourite teacher or where he went on family holidays. Instead, he tells me about the willow warbler's nest he found in the bank of an overgrown ditch and the grey partridge's nest with 12 pale olive eggs concealed in a patch of nettles at the edge of a wood. A treasured collection of oological memories that he's been adding to over the past 20 years.

These days, during the breeding season, my walks with Dad are stealthy affairs. His techniques involve dipping in and out of copses and circling patches of scrub. Along the way, I'm taught the tricks of the trade. I learn 'cold searching' first. This method, sometimes known in the business as 'legging', involves looking for nests in suitable locations. We crouch, then tilt our heads to angle along a sightline, or balance on tiptoe to peer deep into the bushes looking for clues – a dense clump of leaves (perhaps a wren's nest), a scribble of sticks (woodpigeon) or a stray curl of dried grass suggesting a woven nest further in (blackbird). It takes me a while to get my eye in, then the visual anomalies start to snag. I spot a tangle of twigs and moss – a dunnock's nest at head height just off the path, awkward to get to through the prickly hawthorn but Dad manages to manoeuvre his telescopic mirror to the correct angle and it reveals three light-blue eggs at the base of a grassy rootlet bowl.

Dad records the nest on his phone. Later, he'll transfer the data onto the British Trust for Ornithology (BTO) Nest Record Scheme – he's progressed in the last 60 years from short-trousered tree-climber to experienced nest recorder. He'll return to the dunnock's nest once a week for the next month or so to record progress and ring the nestlings once they're old enough.

Further along the scrubby hedge Dad takes me through another nest-location tactic: 'watching back', sometimes known by the technical term 'arsing'. Wrens are an ideal species to watch back, as their nests are often tucked deep in the vegetation, but they can be located by the exceedingly complex technique of sitting on your arse, watching birds flying past with nest material or insects for their young. Once you notice this telltale behaviour, you can move to 'hot searching' to pinpoint the exact location, tapping the vegetation gently if it's not possible to see the nest so any sitting bird is alerted and can move off until you're done.

Finding nests without disturbing the birds relies on a good knowledge of different species. Birds are more likely to abandon the nest if they're disturbed when they don't have eggs or young (before they've made much investment in the nesting attempt). Chaffinches and greenfinches are particularly prone to deserting if interrupted at this stage, so we'll retreat if we see them with nest material. Similar caution is necessary when recording the nests of *Sylvia* warblers like blackcap and whitethroat, and other open-nesters such as dunnock, blackbird and song thrush. Any disturbance risks triggering more mature chicks' anti-predator response, causing them to explode off the nest if they're startled. We also avoid too much disturbance of the vegetation so as not to alert predators to the presence of the nests.

Dad has to walk carefully in some areas to avoid damaging nests on or close to the ground. Both willow warblers and chiffchaffs build domed nests from grass, moss and leaves. Willow warbler nests are always on the ground, while chiffchaffs build off the ground (even if by only a few centimetres). Over the years, he's found chiffchaff nests in nettles, brambles and sedges, and a willow warbler's nest in a clump of grass at the base of a hawthorn sapling. He's also monitored many other species, including reed bunting, whitethroat, reed warbler and a linnet's nest with four pale eggs speckled with purple. But in Dad's mind, nothing surpasses the Cetti's warbler.

He tells me about his find as we walk towards the nest site and he's as excited as I've ever seen him, practically rubbing his hands together with glee. "Last month, I thought I was monitoring six blackcap nests – two with eggs, one lined and ready for eggs and the rest unfinished," he tells me. "The lined one was over here in a dense patch of scrub. It's visible, but not easy to see." Dad gets out his mirror-on-a-stick. "When I came back last week and looked in the nest, I was amazed to see three beautiful red eggs. Not a blackcap. A Cetti's warbler's nest!" I can feel my own excitement building in response to his. Many of the nests we've found today have been predated and I'm desperately hoping this one will still contain eggs.

"It's a Schedule 1 species," he says, "so I couldn't visit again without permission. I got in touch with the BTO and they sent me a licence, so now I can carry on monitoring." He inserts his mirror into the brambles and, to his delight, it reveals four eggs – one more than last week. They're due to hatch in around ten days. The eggs are astonishing. Glorious terracotta-red with a polished sheen as if they've been buffed to liquid perfection by the adult's breast. And, with only 20–30 Cetti's warbler nestlings ringed most years in the UK, Dad is over the moon at the prospect of ringing the chicks in a couple of weeks.

Although the purpose of our visit is to collect scientific data and our activities are all legal and licensed, something about the process still feels a tad illicit. Perhaps it's the subterfuge and specialist knowledge required or the way Dad is passing on skills partly gleaned from his early birdnesting days. Whatever the reason, I know we're unlikely to have a negative impact on the birds. The BTO website explains that provided their guidelines are followed 'extensive reviews of scientific studies... indicate that visits to solitary nesting birds, particularly passerines, have little or no significant effect on the outcome of the breeding attempt'. And the Nest Record Scheme relies heavily on the work of volunteers like Dad to compile the data. All his nest records, together with his Wetland Bird Survey results, ringing records and breeding bird surveys, help inform conservation decisions such as which species will be added to the Birds of Conservation Concern Red List, a roll-call that now includes an eye-watering 73 of the UK's 245 bird species. These days, Dad's close encounters with nesting birds have a scientific purpose. But as a small boy, he just liked collecting the eggs.

In March 1972, nearly a year after getting married, my parents moved out of their rented flat and bought a 50-metre garden in Nuneaton for £5,000. It came with a three-bed semi. The top garden was mostly lawn, with a concrete path leading down the middle. At the end of the lawn stood an old cedar-wood greenhouse. The bottom section of the garden had been used as an allotment and was split into four transverse strips. The first contained James Grieve and Bramley apple trees, a peach tree and gooseberry bushes. Immediately behind this strip was the vegetable plot split into three beds separated by grass paths. Couch grass and clubroot were rife. In one of the overgrown veg beds, the previous owners had left a row of parsnips. When Dad went to investigate, the top growth reached up to his nose.

He was thrilled with his first garden. He built a compost bin, a new aluminium greenhouse and the geometrically challenged garage (he did get the car in once, but tells me getting it out was a nightmare), then set about growing his own fruit and veg. No doubt, by the summer, our garden would have been full of massive leeks, wormy carrots and stringy runner beans – vegetable familiars that I recall with a shudder. But there would also have been strawberries, peas, lettuce, kohlrabi, tomatoes, cucumbers and radishes. In later years, I remember Dad's vegetable beds as untidily productive, our kitchen lined with bowls of home-grown fruit and stewed apple, freezers packed with bags of blanched veg. It never occurred to me to question the time he spent in the garden while the plaster showed through in bare strips on our lounge walls. His priorities seemed – still seem – to make sense. Why spend precious time inside when you could be planting in the borders or watching wrens in the reedbeds?

Over the next few months, my parents settled into their new life. They joined the local RSPB group and made friends in the birding community. Coventry was a hub of ornithological activity, home to one of the new members' groups co-ordinated by RSPB Regional Organiser, Trevor Gunton. The first group (North East London, now known as Epping Forest) was established in 1969 and by October of that year there were plans afoot to set up a local group in Coventry. They organised their first trip – to Eyebrook Reservoir near Corby to watch winter ducks – in mid-December. By the following year, the Coventry group were part of a regional film network, showing RSPB wildlife films and raising money for the society. They were one of the most active and progressive local groups, and their first film presentation of *The Winged Aristocrats* (about Europe's birds of prey, including peregrine falcon and snowy owl) and *Birds of the Grey Wind* (focusing on bird life in Northern Ireland) attracted an audience of over a thousand people.

By the RSPB's Centenary Year in 1989, there were 176 members' groups running nearly 250 annual film shows. They raised thousands of pounds, recruited hundreds of new members and provided a forum for people to get together to share their love of birds. Dad volunteered to be secretary of the Coventry group and co-ordinated a programme of talks by leading ornithologists like Peter Conder, Director of the RSPB. Peter gave a talk on the wheatear, a bird about which he'd write a monograph 14 years later, based on 40 years of observation and his colour-ringing studies on Skokholm, an island off the Pembrokeshire coast. It was the first time my dad had heard the earthy etymology of this attractive chat, its common name derived from the Old English for 'white arse' referring to the white rump, revealed when the bird takes flight.

Field trips were another enjoyable part of the group's activities. The itinerary in the early 70s took in salubrious locations like Wisbech Sewage Works, nearby Brandon Marshes and Ynys-hir to the south of Snowdonia, and also included a dawn chorus visit to Salcey Forest in Northamptonshire. Then, in May 1974, Mum and Dad spread their wings on a trip to Norway with friends from the group. Led by two of the Coventry RSPB founders, Brian and Janet Wright, they spent a month travelling round the Arctic coast. Brian was the birdbrain of the expedition, keeper of their ambitious tick list. Species in his sights included snowy owls, red-necked phalaropes, white-tailed eagles and wood sandpipers.

I get out my parents' old albums and squint at the 35mm slides through an 8x magnifier loupe, which adds to the vintage feel of browsing images from almost half a century ago. Holding slides up to the light, I walk my eye across snowy plateaus in the Saltfjellet mountain range, north of the Arctic Circle; I gaze up torrenting waterfalls and peer into glassy fjords. I wonder what impact these sheer landscapes had on my parents and their friends, fresh from birding in Midland marshes and sewage works in the fens.

After a series of wild unpeopled vistas, an image of my parents sitting on deckchairs outside their cabin in the Dovrefjell mountains takes me by surprise. Mum looks tanned and happy in a lavender roll-necked sweater, lying back with her eyes closed, hands interlaced across her stomach. Dad's grinning at the photographer, his black hair all overgrown and bushy, binoculars on his lap. I grin back at him, amused by the reappearance of his infamous horseshoe moustache. Curving down round the corners of his upturned mouth, the impressive 'pipes' give him the look of a shaggy cowboy. For my first decade that majestic moustache was my dad. It framed him. It was part of him and, by association, part of me. Then, one morning when I was ten – without warning – Dad shaved it off. I was inconsolable. It was a betrayal. How could he still be my dad without his moustache? Now the old photos make me chortle. Thank God he got rid of it before I became a teenager. Life's hard enough without your dad impersonating a hairy biker or 1970s porn star.

I scan the slides for more amusement at his expense, but this sunny scene is the only appearance of Dad and his moustache.

The rest of the time he's behind the camera, attempting to record the landscape and its birds. The quality of his images reveals how far his equipment and techniques have come over the past five decades. In one slide I can see a dry grassy hollow and what might be a couple of dark blurry eggs, but Dad has to identify them for me as belonging to a golden plover. Several shots focus on an uninspiring rocky clifftop. Then I spot a white face poking out, the carnival colours of a puffin's bill all washed out in the grimy light. In another, a female eider duck is just visible in a ramshackle wooden shelter near the top of a cliff. I presume she's sitting on eggs.

Birding was very much a shared passion for my parents, and the holiday acted as a tonic for Mum. She loved their helicopter trip to the island of Røst in the Lofoten archipelago in search of wading birds like the red-necked phalarope. Dad's photograph of this delicate bird is of a tiny speck making ripples in a boggy pool. Known in Norway as the *svømmesnipe*, or swimming snipe, the phalarope spins round in circles churning up invertebrates, and Mum and Dad had superb views of this particular individual. But its slender coppery neck and white throat are barely visible in the photograph, its sooty head swallowed by the grey reflections of the mountains. It seems likely that other slides record equally intimate encounters but, if so, the details are too small to be seen. On their return, frustrated with the poor quality of the developed images, Dad bought his first proper camera for wildlife photography – the Praktica L with Vivitar 200mm telephoto lens.

Though she found their expeditions exciting, Mum struggled to keep up with the others as they crossed the Arctic tundra and slogged through the mires. Brian would apologise for the terrain he'd led them into, all "bog and ack" he'd say when he saw her trudging behind the group. He'd lag at the rear to keep her company, teaching her to walk uphill with a slight forward lean at the ankles. He promised her the sight of a *snøugle* for her twenty-fourth birthday, but the snowy owls in the Børgefjell mountains were not obliging and they remained an unticked birthday dream. In one of the images, Mum walks with Brian and Janet along a snowy slope, all three with binoculars at the ready. They look young and keen, Brian with his orange waterproof jacket slung over his pack. He'd bought it before they left, convinced it would camouflage him against the lichen-covered rocks. The others ribbed him mercilessly. Even in late May, the ground was still tucked under a white winter duvet, awaiting the summer melt. He stuck out like an orange sore thumb against the pristine snow and silver limbs of the leafless mountain birches.

My parents made lasting friendships on the Norway trip. They continued to birdwatch with Brian and Janet, keeping in touch when we moved to Cheshire eight years later. Then, in late November 1984, the Wrights left for a once-in-a-lifetime trip to The Gambia. The highlight of their holiday was to be a birding excursion along the River Gambia on the six-deck MV *Lady Chilel Jawara*. Boarding on the afternoon of Tuesday 4 December, they joined the 73 Gambian deck passengers and 23 other British birders hoping to see iconic species like Egyptian plover and the elusive African finfoot. The 500-mile round trip set out from the capital, Banjul, on the Atlantic coast, sailed upstream to Basse, the most easterly main town in the country, before returning to Banjul later in the week. Only, on this voyage, the *Lady Chilel Jawara* did not return.

On the morning of Friday 7 December, the ship capsized and sank off Devil Point, a bend in the river near the village of Balingho. Dave Farrow, another British birder on the trip, wrote about the moment – at 10.10 a.m. – when the ship began to list to port. As the right-hand side of the boat lifted up above him, passengers clung to the handrail by their fingertips, ending up hanging parallel to the deck. Tumbling into the river when the boat turned over, he managed to stay clear of the hull and grab onto a gas canister. The current started to carry him downstream and he was towed back to the boat by one of his companions. They climbed onto the upturned hull to join the other survivors and wait for help.

Six hours later, they were relieved to see the roll-on roll-off ferry approaching the wreck to take them to a jetty a couple of miles upstream. Solid ground, at last. But not all the passengers made it off the river that day. A young Gambian girl drowned, along with three birders from Coventry: Jon Baldwin, a voluntary warden at Brandon Marsh Reserve, and Brian and Janet Wright. Janet was knocked unconscious as the boat turned over, and she drowned in the river. Brian's body was never found. I remember eating dinner at the kitchen table just before we left for the Christingle Service and hearing about the Gambian disaster on the news; the look on my mum's face; the sadness that followed. They'd been to stay with us just three weeks earlier. Mum told me later that it was tragic but also somehow right that they'd gone down together. They had been so much in love, she said, that neither would have wanted to go on without the other.

Although Mum struggled to keep up in Norway, she assumed it was as a result of her fluctuating health as she knew nothing about energy-limiting conditions at that time. It wasn't until they got home that she realised she was pregnant. Surprisingly, as the months went by, her health began to improve. She had increased energy levels and a sense of wellbeing that lasted throughout the second and third trimesters. Pregnancy suits the women in my family. Like Mum's, my pregnancies were fairly straightforward, if you ignore a few weeks of morning sickness in the first trimester. If we encounter problems, they tend to set in postpartum.

When my second child – a daughter – was born after 27 hours of labour, I couldn't work out whether today was actually today or if it was still yesterday. All I knew was I'd been at it a sod of a long time and I was relieved to have managed a successful vaginal birth after my previous caesarean. We'd done it together, this little bairn and me. And here she was, lying against my chest – my scrunched-up daughter, her bloodied head and tiny button nose, that pixie profile I'd fallen in love with at my 12-week scan.

Her body was intimate, warm, near at hand; mine felt torn and far away. When the midwives stitched me up the first time, I watched remotely, but when the senior midwife came in and repeated the process considerably less gently, declaring she could still see a hole, the scene took on a kind of grotesque surrealism. Only my lips felt awake, cracked and swollen into painful consciousness from hours dragging on gas and air. Me, my lips and the bairn, lying on bedsheets drenched with blood from our newly qualified midwife's unsuccessful attempt to insert the cannula. We'd joked the room looked like the aftermath of a massacre before I'd even started and my husband hid behind a screen in the corner for a while to avoid fainting and requiring medical attention himself.

I've retained only a few fragments of the blurry days that followed. In some I'm rainbow-surfing above a sky-land which I picture now, nearly a decade later, as looking rather like Laputa, the floating island that Gulliver visits on his travels. Perhaps the psychedelic colours that illuminate the clouds are rays of light shattered by the adamantine ground below or – and I'm willing to accept this is the more likely scenario – they are the leftover reflections of the morphine I begged for and eventually received during the final few hours of labour.

Another memory points downwards and inwards. I'm in the kitchen, only a day or so after giving birth, cradling my daughter in my arms and oh! she is perfect, so soft and present, and so completely and utterly mine. I hold her tightly against my chest and when my husband comes in to check if we need anything, for a second, I don't register it's him. I pull back into the corner between the cupboards and fold myself around her. All I know in that moment is that this new baby is mine and no one else can have her.

This feeling passed quickly enough and within days she was being cuddled by family and friends while I looked on, happy and grateful for the caring circle of people who would support her as she grew. Looking back now, my strength of feeling in the kitchen surprises me. I'm pleased when my kids spend time with other people; it's good for their development and strengthens family relationships. But at that moment I had such a deep sense that we two were still one. Passing her over for cuddles, even to my husband, would have been tantamount to wrenching out my heart and giving it away. I think her birth was a righting of sorts, the creation of a healing bond.

My birth was a far swifter, though no less painful affair. On Valentine's Day 1975, the day P. G. Wodehouse died aged 93 and a bomb was discovered at Venserpolder station in Amsterdam, my dad was busy chatting to the midwife about the Rugby League World Cup. He'd been sent away earlier to get a bite to eat as my shoulder was stuck in the birth canal and I didn't appear to be going anywhere. Then I started to move, fast, and Dad was summoned back in. The room was stuffy and he was soon regretting the fish and chips he'd eaten in the hospital canteen. He began to feel decidedly sick. Rugby was a good distraction to keep his mind off the oppressive atmosphere and my imminent birth.

Rather than being given morphine as I was when giving birth, Mum was offered only gas and air, which didn't work, and the dreadful pain from my lodged shoulder sent her body into shock. I was born just half an hour later at 20 minutes to midnight. It seems Dad retained both his dinner and his sense of humour, commenting that my head was shaped just like a rugby ball, but my shoulder had done Mum lasting damage.

She spent the first few weeks of my life unable to get out of bed, barely functioning, battling pain, debilitating exhaustion and severe postnatal depression. Unsurprisingly in these circumstances, she found it impossible to bond with me. When she looked at me, she explained recently, she felt nothing but misery. I find it upsetting to imagine those days. Mum plunged back into illness, struggling to meet a newborn's needs without the hormonal support of the mother–child bond that I found came so easily with my children. Despite her chronic illness and postnatal depression, Mum had no way to access help from any support services. Nothing was in place for a woman considered a malingerer. Granny called in some days, willing to do what she could, though she didn't really understand what was wrong, but much of the time Mum had no option but to attempt to look after me on her own. She found my crying difficult to cope with. On one occasion, she threw me in my cot and took herself off down the bottom of the garden. She was afraid, if she'd stayed with me, she would have hurt me. Mum recalls crawling across the floor one afternoon when I was a few months old to get me a banana for my lunch because she could not walk. If there was a fire, she thought, she would not be able to get us out.

I too had times soon after my first child was born, before I received my diagnosis, when I felt so exhausted and mentally low that it was tough to keep going but, however ill I felt, I'd still have been able to pick up my baby and run for the door if I'd seen flames. I feel for Mum struggling across that carpet and wish I'd been there, other than in my newly arrived state, to offer her a shoulder to lean on. When she plucked up the courage to ask for help, the health visitors told her it was all in her head. Of course they did. The age-old story trotted out when a woman feels pain or finds herself close to the edge.

"Don't make a fuss."
"Pull yourself together."
"Don't be so dramatic."

This was the mid-70s, of course. A different era. And yet I wonder how much has really changed. You don't have to go far, even today, to come across attitudes that trivialise women's pain. I was chatting to an older guy only the other day at the end of a birding session. He mentioned a friend who'd recently had Covid and, having expressed sympathy for his friend's suffering, added, as if for emphasis: "And when a man says he's in real pain, it must be bad."

I wondered about the corollary to this. When a woman says she's in real pain, it's not actually that bad? Because women are moaners? Because we exaggerate the levels of pain we experience? Perhaps he felt men suffer in stoical silence until pain becomes unbearable, whereas women whimper at the first intimation of discomfort. Menstrual cramps and childbirth: common causes of pain that women are simply expected to deal with. Preferably without complaint. So I kept my silence. After all, I didn't know him very well. But if you'd been standing in my shoes, you'd have heard me screaming inside.

Many scientific studies back up the anecdotes. Reports on medical treatments offered for pain suggest prescription decisions are partly determined by gender. Women in pain tend to be left waiting longer in A & E before being treated and are less likely to be given analgesia than men. Evidence shows this is even more likely with women in minoritised ethnic groups, especially in childbirth. There are also certain conditions, often affecting only women, that are notoriously poorly diagnosed and treated, despite the potential for causing severe pain, anxiety and depression over many years. Endometriosis is one such condition. In 2020, according to a survey by Endometriosis UK, it took an average of eight years in the UK from the onset of symptoms to receiving a diagnosis. By 2023 the wait time had risen to eight years and ten months, and 78 per cent of those who were subsequently diagnosed with endometriosis had been told by one or more doctors that they were making a fuss about nothing or something similar. And it isn't as though endometriosis is a rare condition; in fact, it affects 10 per cent of women of reproductive age.

I was lucky, in some respects. Last year when I began to experience almost constant pelvic pain, my GP was sympathetic. She referred me to the gynaecology department at my local hospital and within a couple of months a transvaginal ultrasound revealed I had adenomyosis, a condition related to endometriosis. In both cases, tissue similar to that in the lining of the womb starts to grow in the wrong place. In endometriosis it often develops in areas such as the ovaries and fallopian tubes; with adenomyosis it grows deep within the muscle of the womb, causing uterine swelling and pain. Like endometriosis, adenomyosis is thought to affect around one in ten women of reproductive age, but the condition has only recently been given its own page on the NHS website. And while I feel fortunate that my diagnosis was swift and will, I hope, lead to effective pain relief in the near future, I've started to look back and wonder.

I remember little of my time at sixth form college, but I can close my eyes and transport myself in an instant to the girls' toilets where I fought to overcome my period pain one truly miserable morning. The aching in my abdomen as I write, caused by my as-yet-untreated adenomyosis, makes it easy to reach back and inhabit my teenage pain. I'm huddled up over my knees on the loo seat, hoping the girls in the other cubicles won't notice the moaning noises I can't stop making. I've taken a Feminax but the paracetamol- and codeine-based pill has had no discernible effect on the cramps that grip my abdomen and spill over into my back, groin and legs. I'm wondering if it would be physically possible to knock myself unconscious, whether I could strike hard enough to put myself out of my own misery.

Clenched there, rocking, I begin to fantasise about hitting myself over the head with a vase. Why I reached for such a breakable implement, I've no idea. Perhaps dramatic pain required a dramatic solution. Of course, I never went through with it. Dramatic scenes weren't really my strong point and in the outside world we were taught that pain was just a normal part of a girl's life, another step on what I considered the loathsome path to becoming a woman. But inside, when the monthly cramps came, I felt real despair. Instead of useless pills, I wished for oblivion.

I was in my twenties before I decided this wasn't normal. My GP prescribed mefenamic acid (which I nicknamed the 'hit-and-miss' pill) but didn't investigate the cause. Occasionally I'd hit the sweet spot, swallowing the tablet in that random half-hour window when it seemed to kick in as it should, blocking the enzymes creating inflammation and pain. Then I'd luxuriate in hours of pure relief. But the acid pill was more miss than hit and I had only one chance to score. I had no idea why it didn't always work. If I didn't take it soon enough after the pain began, it had no effect whatsoever. Every unsuccessful month I was left to devise my own distractions from the pain – hours walking round my room in the middle of the night, futile leg rotations lying on my side in bed, endless lengths of the swimming pool. "Exercise relieves the discomfort," they told me. "Like hell it does," I should have replied.

Quite why I didn't go back to the doctor to ask why the medication was so often useless, I don't know. I think I felt I'd be blamed and ignored. I wish I'd had the confidence to turn my pain inside out and externalise the internal screaming. Perhaps then I'd have asked for and been offered help. If I'd had an ultrasound or MRI scan in those early days, it might have revealed a womb already enlarged with invasive tissue. At my last appointment, the consultant told me new research now suggests many women with adenomyosis may have had it for many years. More likely though, I'd have been sent away with a flea in my ear and different, but equally ineffectual, painkillers.

Like me and so many women before me, Mum received no validation for her physical or mental pain in those months following my birth; no hand was extended to pull her back from the brink. She simply faced denial. Denial which she accepted without question. Decades of ill health without medical support or diagnosis had habituated her to systematic disbelief and gaslighting. Without any explanation for her depression and exhaustion, she simply thought this was the way everyone felt after having a baby. Presumably other people just tried harder to cope – a conclusion I'd come to myself, many years later, not realising this self-doubt ran through my female line like a necrosis that devours you from within.

For my parents, struggling with a newborn baby and Mum's undiagnosed illness and postnatal depression, the natural world was a vital source of comfort and distraction. More importantly for Mum, whose ability to walk any distance was often restricted, it was accessible just outside the back door. One night at the washing up, Dad spotted a moth on the outside of the kitchen window. He went to take a look, not expecting much. Moths were dull. Little brown jobs. But not this one. When it was at rest with its wings folded, he could see grey-brown patches finely marked with loops and lines, divided by metallic sections where the wing seemed touched with greenish gold leaf. Blown away by its beauty, he caught it in an empty jam jar and took it up to Mum. It lifted her mood for a while and identifying moths in bed together soon became a regular nocturnal affair. Dad bought the two-volume *The Moths of the British Isles* and discovered their gilded visitor was a burnished brass – one of the noctuid (from the Latin for 'night owl'), or owlet, moths – so called because of the way their eyes reflect light in the darkness.

Dad's interest was piqued and it wasn't long before he was (in Mum's words) a fully formed "moth nerd". She was a new mother and now a new moth-er – his assistant 'nerd-in-training' – sitting up with him late into the night, leafing through the field guides now stacked on the shelf behind me. My parents' interest in moths gave them a shared focus, their two heads bent together over the bed as they tried to identify each new species. Later, they'd buy a cheap 20-watt Heath trap (a simple rectangular box with a funnel and a small fluorescent tube) and, as their ID skills improved, Dad recorded the details of more than 150 species on meticulous graphs and spreadsheets. So the moths and the months passed and, by the time I was one and a half, Mum had recovered from her postnatal depression. For a while, at least, life returned to normal. Then, in spring 1977, she discovered she was pregnant again.

My brother and I were both the subjects of mother-and-baby studies during the first year of our lives. My notes are long gone, but Stephen still has his. A section at the beginning of his file refers to my baby study, which had been undertaken a couple of years earlier by a young woman called Lesley for her CSE Childcare Examination. I wonder what Lesley saw, or thought she saw, when she observed me and my parents during this time.

Stephen's report, written by a young woman on a nursery nursing course at college, includes nearly 50 pages of notes covering a period from a few weeks before his birth until his first birthday. It paints an idyllic picture of our 'very close and loving' family unit, happily awaiting the arrival of the new baby. I appear on the margins at 'two years of age... a very intelligent little girl with a marvellous imagination and intense curiosity.' I was keen on the idea of a sibling and asked endless questions. The notes say I had a new book about babies. I guess it would have given me a lot to think about.

Early October, 1977
At this stage, the report suggests that all is well. Grandma is set to look after me while Mum is in hospital; the baby box, bottles, sterilising unit, pram and cot are on standby and the maternity grant has arrived. Reading this spick and span section of the report, I'm reminded of the old *Janet and John* books. I imagine myself decked out in a pastel frock with ribbons in my hair, sitting on a fence or playing demurely with a rag doll; Mum impressively coiffured, perhaps handing round drinks; Dad besuited, arriving home from work, a natty fedora in his hand. Of course, these images belong to an earlier era. Mum coiffured?

Dad in a fedora? What ridiculous notions! Janet and John were already 30 years past their childhoods when I was learning to read at the end of the 70s. But initially the baby study has a whiff of utopian family life about it.

Wednesday 26 October
Stephen's delivery is fairly straightforward. Easier than my birth, though he is born with the cord wrapped round his neck twice and the nurses have to work quickly to cut him free before it strangles him.

Sunday 30 October
Mum is noted as having slight depression, which has disappeared by the end of the first week.

Tuesday 22 November
For the first four weeks, mother and baby are well. Everyone is happy. I accept my brother right from the start. When he's propped up on the settee after a feed, I walk up to him, fling my arms around him and smother him in kisses. Photographs show us surrounded by the décor of the decade taste forgot, sat on a brown settee with orange flecks (the other settee in the room was orange with brown stripes), me in denim dungarees looking pensively at the camera, my Ladybird Book *Animals, Birds and Plants of the Bible* on my lap. Stephen is propped up against orange velour cushions.

9 a.m., Friday 2 December
Over the past week, Stephen's feeding has deteriorated. His tendency to bring back milk develops into projectile vomiting

and he is rushed to hospital. A surgeon diagnoses congenital pyloric stenosis, a condition in babies where the opening between the stomach and small intestine narrows and can become blocked. He is due to have the Ramstedt's operation that afternoon to repair his pyloric muscle, but ends up waiting until the evening as he needs a blood transfusion.

9 p.m., Friday 2 December
After the operation, the scalp vein drip on Stephen's shaved head begins to leak. Fluid pools in his tissues. His face swells to a grotesque size. None of the hospital staff notice. It isn't until my parents visit the ward that they see his face and call the nurses in panic. The drip is removed. The bloating subsides.

Sunday 4 December
Stephen's stomach wound ruptures. He has to have his sutures replaced under general anaesthetic.

Friday 9 December
Stephen is discharged at seven weeks old, wearing a baby girl's dress. There are no boys' clothes small enough for him. He weighs just 6 pounds 8 ounces. Once at home, he goes from strength to strength, putting on up to half a pound a day, though he is not the contented baby he was prior to the operation. But the damage to Mum's precarious postnatal health has been done. She believes the hospital have been negligent and loses any remaining faith in the medical profession. Struggling along silently, she hides her depression from almost everyone, including health visitors and doctors.

January 1978

Stephen is now three months old and, reading the baby study, you'd think everything is going swimmingly. Both Mum's and Stephen's check-ups show them to be in good health and the report describes a happy and contented little boy with a much more relaxed mother.

Early April

Bottling up her emotions is not a long-term solution and Mum can't keep up the pretence any longer. She collapses again. The report explains that this new mental health crisis is a result of her suppressing her despair and confirms she is now very ill, suffering from severe depression. The doctor prescribes antidepressants and sleeping pills. They don't help. Mum is unable to get out of bed for six weeks and has periods of almost complete paralysis, each one lasting up to five days. She describes the symptoms as being like brain flu, bones like shells, rope-bound, ground-down. During this, her worst period, she's still offered no explanation for her illness by the midwives or doctors. She has been told often enough that it is all in her head. By this point, Mum is convinced that she is going mad.

By the middle of April, Dad had hardly been at work for weeks. Mum was unable to look after us and the doctor arranged for a psychiatrist to assess the situation. On the day of the visit, my parents were hoping for understanding and support. But the psychiatrist spoke almost exclusively to my dad, as if my mum's exhaustion and depression, and perhaps her gender, rendered her incapable of making her own decisions. His only words to Mum were to tell her that she needed to be admitted to a psychiatric ward. He didn't believe my dad could look after a three-year-old and a baby on his own, so told him we needed to go into care. His visit compounded Mum's overactive sense of guilt. Not only was she struggling with an undiagnosed illness, which people had convinced her was all in her head, but now she felt she'd failed to look after her children properly. In the days following the psychiatrist's visit, our family faced being torn apart by a medical system entrenched in scepticism, intolerance and sexism.

With our future at stake, Dad decided to resign from his job as an electrical engineer. But when he offered his resignation, it was rejected. Instead, he was given three months' paid leave. My grandma came to stay for a few weeks and arrangements were made for me to start morning nursery at the local primary school, even though I was only three years and two months – six months younger than the other children. Every morning, my mum would say "See you later, alligator," and I'd reply "In a while, crocodile." Then Grandma would walk me to school. Stephen's baby report says I liked nursery. I enjoyed the extra stimulation and the opportunity to play with other children. Yet, despite the extra help, Mum continued to have bouts of severe depression. Dad told me, years later, that he had considered moving out and asking Mum for a divorce. By this point, it had all become too much for him.

We were lucky that our health visitor, who'd also helped after my birth, believed Mum and kept telling her something was physically wrong. She said she'd keep coming every day until we got sorted, and she never gave up on us. It was on her suggestion that Mum visited a consultant for a second opinion. Without the persistence of this caring health visitor, our lives would have taken a very different turn. As it was, the consultation led to a referral to Dr Patrick Kingsley, a renowned practitioner of complementary medicine. Dr Kingsley diagnosed Mum with myalgic encephalomyelitis (a debilitating multisystem neurological condition now commonly referred to as ME/CFS) and offered to treat her.

Finally, she had a diagnosis. And Dad decided to stay. Mum had been so good to him, he thought. And they had the garden and the garage, the birds and the moths – those nocturnal sessions bonding over scalloped hazels, clouded borders and sallow kittens. Late in the evening, after my brother and I were in bed, their thoughts would turn to the trap. It was their time together. The dark time. Illuminated by enigmatic creatures of the night. The intricate wing markings, often so similar on different species, required close examination. I can imagine them, heads nearly touching as they savoured the features of a gem like the sallow kitten moth. Its downy head and legs soft as eiderdown, its white folded forewings speckled with orange and charcoal like rusted iron ore, finished with a border of dark dots. Absorbed in the infinite wonders of the natural world, Dad was distracted from his worries and Mum forgot her feelings of guilt and inadequacy. Moths brought my parents together physically and emotionally. Looking forward to the night's treasures gave them the gift of hope.

Now, with nearly 50 years' hindsight, I can see there were many reasons why we made it through this difficult time as a family. But my parents' shared love of the natural world played a key role in strengthening their relationship. It offered a regular dose of joy when despair and divorce were near at hand. With my dad standing by her, and certain now that her health problems were caused by a physical illness, my mum decided to ignore the psychiatrist's advice. She stayed at home and we stayed with her. Our family unit remained intact.

Watcher in
the Shadows

Plunged, nose first, into a morning of cold, sharp smells. Dad and I are decorating my brother's bedroom and we're taking a break. We've not been in our new house long. I'm seven or eight and, apart from the bombweed, this is my earliest memory. The air is turps, paint, dust, concrete floors. I'm sat on the bottom rung of the step ladder in the middle of the boxroom, my new book *Ich Bin Klein, Du Bist Gross* open on my lap. Dad is teaching me German. I love it when he reads to me. Love the cheerful pictures in my book, the unfamiliar sticky sounds of the words. Love knowing that Dad will always be there. Solid and safe. Bristly. Smelling of Imperial Leather. Forever *Gross* to my *Klein*.

When we're in the garden, Dad works alone and I potter after him, first with buckets and sticks, later with saws and files, messing about with wood, or with books and notepads, reading and studying. I pick strawberries, raspberries and peas, flicking off the slugs, winkling out pea moth caterpillars and raspberry beetle larvae. Learn to cut the lawn with a cantankerous petrol mower, so bad-tempered it needs my dad's superhuman strength to start the engine 'third time lucky'. We set up a society in our garden shed with badges, passwords and a spy ring, but we're hampered by a frustrating lack of local villains or baffling crimes to solve. Instead, we focus on other top-secret activities, so confidential I can't let on or I'd have to kill you.

I get to know the wild life in our wild garden. I join the Young Ornithologists' Club and learn to identify the birds that visit the wooden bird table that Dad built. The peanuts attract coal tits, greenfinches and a nuthatch, which I no doubt tick off in my *I-Spy Birds* book. Occasionally, a green woodpecker comes an-anting on the patio, and just once we have fleeting views of a redstart in the apple trees. I sketch some bivalve shells I've fished out of Tatton Mere, noting their diameter (4.5 centimetres), circumference (9 centimetres), weight (6 grams) and age – by counting the shell rings as you would a tree (21 years). I write poems about autumn and wonder what it would feel like to be a raindrop. I watch our soppy cat Tiger chase a rabbit across the lawn, only to reappear a moment later pursued by the rabbit. He leaps in the air to swallow bees that somehow don't sting him and pats frogs from paw to paw, letting them go only when he's had his fill of friendly prodding.

One day it appears he's not been so friendly with a field vole. I put its cold, squashed body on the windowsill and go to find my brother to show him before I bury it, but when we return ten minutes later, the vole has vanished. I watch black garden ants frothing up from their nests under the paving stones in the patio, stubbing out a few with my plimsolls to see how long it takes the undertakers to haul the corpses away for some nefarious purpose or other. The organisation and speed with which they deal with my delinquent interventions fascinates me.

Despite this ant-assassination phase, I always loved animals. Furred or feathered, finned or tentacled, wild or tame. As a little kid, I had big plans to farm garden snails for a living. I figured it would be easy-peasy. The raw materials were simple to find: lettuce leaves, polystyrene SpudULike containers, loo roll tubes and plenty of snail volunteers. We were always encouraged to reuse everything (part of a frugal mindset passed down from grandparents and great-grandparents who had to make every penny count), so when we went into Chester for a treat, I'd squirrel away the yellow takeaway pots once I'd scraped them clean of baked potato, cheese and beans with my plastic knife and fork, and bring them home to wash and repurpose into quality snail accommodation.

I made a makeshift cage like the Rotastak we bought later for our hamsters, joining containers together with toilet roll tubes to make a deluxe complex. The snails obligingly ate the food and crawled through the tubes from room to room while I sat on the patio and watched over my new venture with pride. All went well for a while. Then one morning I went out to check on my livestock only to find they'd rasped a hole through the side of one of the tunnels and escaped. I followed their telltale trails across the paving slabs, but they'd disappeared into the flowerbed. I had to accept that my new business had paid poor dividends. Perhaps snail farming wasn't for me after all.

When I was a teenager, we kept stick insects, fish and mice. I had a hankering for bigger, wilder beasts. I'd lose myself in the glossy images of *BBC Wildlife Magazine*, extracting the pictures to stick on my wall – marine mammals first, then anything to do with birds. My most prized poster was a gigantic whale fluke rising from the sea, leviathan power streaming off it in torrents. I'd close my eyes at night on my glow-in-the-dark constellations – Ursa Minor in the corner, its pan handle reaching out to Polaris, Cassiopeia's elongated 'W' on the ceiling above my head – and open them every morning on that poised fluke.

Sometimes, when a potent mix of adolescent hormones and Mum's illness made it hard to kick-start the day, I'd hoick myself out of bed to the sardonic strains of 'Always Look on the Bright Side of Life'. The lyrics appealed to my teenage sense of humour. Since life was undeniably a piece of shit, I reckoned you might as well laugh about it.

Mum spent long periods in bed when I was in the last couple of years at secondary school and again when I was at sixth form college. Unsurprisingly, these bouts of ill health affected her mentally as well as physically. She was often very down, seeing little hope for improved health in the future. She struggled with the sensory and emotional stimulus of having other people in her room, so going to see her wasn't helpful, and I'd learned as a youngster that trying to cheer her up didn't work either. In fact, it seemed to have the opposite effect. I felt helpless. No one discussed her illness with me, school weren't informed and there was no support for our family. Why would there have been? ME/CFS was an invisible illness, so our suffering was invisible too – to society, school, friends, family, even to ourselves. And since there was no reason for my pain, I suppressed it without realising what I was doing. But things came to a head the day Sam died. It shouldn't have been a shock; after all, the lifespan of a pet mouse is around two years, so there's bound to be considerable murine turnover in anyone's childhood. But that wasn't really the point. Sam, one of my Astrex curly haired mice, had had a lump on her flank near one foreleg for a while and I think we all knew her days were numbered. The morning she died I went into sixth form college as normal, but my distress must have been obvious as I soon found myself in the deputy principal's office – a warm-hearted, formidable woman who was also my English teacher. She had the longest, most beautiful white-blonde hair I'd ever seen, like a grown-up Rapunzel, a romantic Christian name – Cherith – and a sharp enquiring mind. Best of all, she seemed to think I had potential. She ignored the indicators when she drove, which I thought the height of risk-taking sophistication, and lived in a cottage with a fairy-tale garden where I went once for extra tuition. I felt gauche, thrilled, like I was on the cusp of something intoxicating: a life of literature, writing and academic debate. She wrote to me on paper with floral margins. She was everything an intellectual woman should be.

How ridiculous I felt, wailing in her office like some snotty-nosed kid. Sam was *just a mouse,* for God's sake. But her tiny death fractured barriers I didn't even realise I'd erected. If I'd been able to view my internal landscape from a distance, this devastating grief for the death of a pet might have been suggestive – the tip of an iceberg or perhaps the mouth of a volcano, spitting with lava from some molten core of sadness within. As it was, I felt confused by the force of my feelings. Why did it feel like all life was illness and suffering? And how excruciatingly embarrassing it was to show vulnerability and emotion. We buried Sam and I unwittingly patched over my mental cracks. After all, she was just a mouse.

I was sensitised to the effects of Mum's illness from an early age. Although it never quite reached the severity it had during my first three years, she struggled with ongoing energy-limitations, depression and brain fog throughout much of my childhood. Her chronic condition formed part of my subconscious landscape. Waking late on a weekend morning, the rest of the family already up and about, I was adrenaline-primed before my mind had even registered a reason, listening for the raised intonation that might indicate Mum was not feeling well, that I'd need to pick my way through the day with care. Her stress levels were closely linked to her fluctuating health, but I think I felt, as a child, that my actions determined Mum's wellbeing. I grew fearful of upsetting her and making her worse. These feelings remained largely subconscious, so I'd have struggled to tell you why hearing the stress in her voice had such a profound effect on me. But even now, if I wake in the morning and hear the children downstairs before I'm fully present, my chest feels tight. I'm on hold in the pit of my stomach until their high voices resolve into laughter, then I realise they're just playing games and I'm not in my childhood bedroom. I rouse myself and find I can breathe out again.

Coming back from school in the afternoons stirred that same simmering anxiety. The windows of our bungalow acted as a barometer of Mum's health. If the curtains were still closed, my heart would sink. The rooms would be colourless and cold, dinner unprepared, and I'd find Mum in bed, physically present but emotionally far, far away. Such periods surfaced intermittently and unpredictably. Dad recalls similar feelings of apprehension when he returned from work late in the evenings. You could read the mood of our house through its windows.

Mum continued to visit the doctor's when she was ill, but mainstream medicine had little to offer beyond blood tests. There you go, her negative results announced after each new appointment, cast-iron proof there's nothing physically wrong with you. It's all in your head. No notion that some illnesses might not be identifiable through bloods, not enough humility to consider some knowledge might still be... unknown. Just the scorn of doctors who hadn't heard of ME/CFS or who did not believe it was real; the gaslighting and disbelief; the lack of interest and the dismissals. Responses that so many people with the condition know only too well. Responses that sent me a clear message. To be less than fully energetic was to be less than. Full stop.

Trying to figure it all out as a child, it seemed clear from the responses of the adults around me that chronic fatigue was seen as embarrassing, overwrought and probably put on. I loved Mum so much and desperately wanted her to be happy and well. But her illness confused me. So I immersed myself in music and books, and tried to ignore the doublethink going on in my head. I wanted to believe she was ill, but also that really, she wasn't. And as no one else seemed sure either, not even my dad, sometimes I doubted her myself. I kept silent about my grubby secret though, unwilling to out myself as a turncoat. What kind of a sick person would suspect their own sick mother?

Complementary medicine offered some support with intravenous vitamin injections, dietary changes and lymph drainage massage, but her core symptoms persisted. I could get my head round some of the treatments she believed in, but other therapies seemed outlandish, even with my rudimentary understanding of science. It felt like someone was being taken for a ride, but I wasn't quite sure who, or by whom. Whatever was going on, I didn't feel we came out well from it. I remember a painful conversation when I was in my early twenties with a friend who told me his opinions about people with ME/CFS – people like Mum – in no uncertain terms. They were time-wasters, conjuring up illness to avoid facing the difficult bits of life. The contempt in his voice made me livid, but I didn't defend her. Somewhere underneath the fury I was ashamed of her, of me, of the inadequacy running through our family.

The aftertaste of shame lingers, even 25 years on. I see now that my feelings of confusion, doubt and embarrassment weren't unnatural; they didn't make me a bad person. But thinking about childhood still picks at the edges of those scabs. I've avoided looking back for so many years, made stories out of everything, except my own life, all to protect that guilty kid from scrutiny. Now, dragged into the open, she starts to panic and follows her gut reaction: kick to the shins, wrench both wrists out of my adult grasp and run for the door. Even you can't force me to share my story, she yells as she flees.

I've always found it hard to talk about my feelings. As a child, there seemed no obvious reason for those times when I felt upset or worried, so I assumed there was something wrong with me. I managed to hide my emotions most of the time, but not always well enough.

"Go to your bedroom," Mum would say, "and don't come out until you're ready to tell me what's wrong." So I'd retreat, wracking my brain for words that would give shape to the numbness inside. Voicing my emotions, even if I'd been able to, would have felt like self-sacrifice – relinquishing control to someone whose reactions could be unpredictable. And who knew where that tale would end? How would I cope if my feelings were twisted, my words hijacked in the service of someone else's need? My solution was to bury them so deeply I forgot they existed. Then I followed my dad's example. I sought refuge in the garden.

Our third-of-an-acre plot in Cheshire came with a 1920s bungalow, set off the busy A49 in a village called Cuddington, en route from Warrington to Chester. From my bedroom, the garden was just a leg-swing over the sill, a head-duck under the casement window, the smallest of hops onto the front path and away. From nurture into nature. In the wild patch at the end of our garden – the rank bit where the grass grew longer and faster than the rest of the lawn and time ran to an incalculable ticking – a towering Scots pine was my runway, eyes turned skywards with apple and book in hand. Up there, surveying the surrounding gardens from my crow's nest (easier to reach than the one Dad shinnied up to as a kid, thanks to a couple of well-placed lower branches), I was invisible and free as a bird. I don't know whether Leonardo da Vinci climbed trees to experience what it might have been like to fly, but I identify with the sentiment that is (almost certainly incorrectly) attributed to him. For there I had always been and there, indeed, I longed to return. Once you've nailed your colours to the mast of a Scots pine as a ten-year-old, you never entirely belong to the earth again.

When I descended, knees and elbows smudged greenish, my hideaway betrayed by indelible algal prints, I'd run to the swing to daub myself streaky blue as my sweaty palms melted the paint off the metal frame. I couldn't get as high on the swing as I could up the tree, but there was movement instead, singing through the dip and rise of my stomach. Swinging made me come alive. I'd tip back my head and smile, whoop again and again because I could, because this rush of movement was joyous and free.

Life beneath me in the garden was busy and vital, colourful and predictable. The raspberries always grew, the rain came, and afterwards the mesembryanthemums opened their candied faces, turning in tandem to worship the sun. I turned my face upwards too, feeling the warmth and a deep sense of connection. Here in the garden I was an active participant in life, a gritty tomboy, self-sufficient and capable. I think I felt, deep down, that if I emulated, even became part of, this more-than-human, intensely alive world that thankfully paid me precious little attention, I might avoid becoming the woman my mother was. Everything seemed to be telling me that women's minds were riddled with emotion, their bodies bred illness and exhaustion. I didn't want my body and mind to spoil like that, so I climbed away from my fears, escaping with my books into the trees.

I spent much of my childhood reading – eclectically, voraciously. I was an inveterate bookworm, devouring stories, consumed by the lives and landscapes therein. To my emotionally hungry child-mind, books were rich and delicious fare, the ultimate comfort food. Not safe exactly, often laced with danger and emotions that felt visceral and real, but once you dug in you could tunnel your way (with that illusion of agency) towards the inevitable resolution, because all the books I read offered some measure of closure. I liked the reassuring plasticity of time in books. Stories were more digestible than real life, less likely to give you heartburn. In the world of fiction, crises were speedily resolved, especially when you read as fast as I did. Nothing lingered like it did in life.

And stories seemed to legitimise intense feelings. Narratives came with their own emotional contours – taking you up to the heights of ecstasy, then plunging you into the slough of despond, and no one monitored or criticised the scale of your feelings along the way. My passageways into these worlds were long and deep like anecic wormholes with an intimate topography that felt mine alone, leading to a nutritious stronghold of stored emotions at their core. Book-worming became a craving, a garrisoning of sorts, like the fantasies I had during pregnancy of eating my way to the centre of a castle-sized chocolate cake and holing up there, gorging myself at leisure to a satiated sweet-and-swollen oblivion. And when you returned to the real world, no one suggested you were making mountains out of molehills if you cried or sulked on the spoil heap of narrative emotion. Unlike real life, it was acceptable to wallow in the aftermath of story.

Fiction was liberating. I found doorways into the wild in the garden of Lucy M. Boston's *Green Knowe*, through the Celtic landscapes of Susan Cooper's *The Dark is Rising* series and the epic vistas of *The Lord of the Rings*. Set in far-off places – Middle Earth, Buckinghamshire, Cornwall, Cambridgeshire – the stories and their settings were exhilarating, but also remote and deeply 'other'. No landscape lured me in with the same immediacy and familiarity as the fields, meres and woods of Alan Garner's *The Weirdstone of Brisingamen*. For starters, the author had nicked my surname. And my dad's identity. Dad was used to being asked "Are you *the* Alan Garner?" "Yes!" he'd always reply. Because, of course, he was. Just not *that* Alan Garner.

The story is set in and around Macclesfield and Alderley Edge (not far from the author's home near Goostrey). Although we lived 25 miles further south, we had friends in Goostrey and cousins in Gawsworth, a village marked on the map in the middle of the book. My home was surrounded by the same boggy, wooded Cheshire terrain through which siblings Susan and Colin travel on their quest to deliver the Weirdstone to the wizard Cadellin Silverbrow. Even when I walked dry-shod to the library or round the corner to visit my school friends, I trod a watery path. Down Mere Lane or Moss Lane, along Forest Road to Blakemere. Behind my house, Cuddington Brook ran into Merlewood Pool, named after an old word for blackbird perhaps, or for the mottled grey-black water. I walked near the pool, sometimes early in the morning, daydreaming or reading, listening to birds I couldn't yet identify.

I learned to canoe in a secluded mere called Petty Pool and hiked in Delamere Forest (the 'forest of the lakes'), a remnant of the twin medieval hunting forests Mara and Mondrem that once stretched 60 square miles across the Cheshire plain. In and around the 2,400 acres of miry forest lie many old bodies of water: Linmer Moss, Hatchmere, Flaxmere Moss, Oakmere, Black Lake, Brackenhurst Bog, Dead Lake, Doolittle Moss. When Susan and Colin walked near Moss Lane in Alderley at the beginning of *The Weirdstone of Brisingamen*, or across to Radnor Mere, listening to the birds that 'sang in the trees, rustled in the thicket, and swam in the many quiet pools', it required little suspension of disbelief on my part to walk with them.

Two years after we moved to Cuddington, in August 1984, Lindow Man was unearthed from a raised mire peat bog on the edge of Wilmslow. Mum took us to see his 2,000-year-old body in Manchester Museum in 1987. I was transfixed. He didn't just die once. One theory was that his skull had been bashed in, then he was garrotted – a sick, leathery word that haunted me for years – and, finally, someone cut his throat. And all this happened thousands of years ago and less than 15 miles away in Lindow Moss, a peat bog like the ones around my home. Mosses and meres. Brooding places. Like Abbots Moss, a *Schwingmoor*, or quaking bog, just down the A49 from my house, where *Sphagnum* mosses grew in floating mats across the water. I walked out over the moss with Dad one day, felt tremors within and beneath me. Dark water and deep time beneath our feet, ready to swallow us whole, like Lindow Man, should we misstep.

When Colin, Susan, Gowther Mossock (a farmer with whom the children were staying) and their companions were offered shelter and safety from pursuit on the floating isle of Angharad Goldenhand on Redesmere, it was easy to imagine living islands that moved. Anything was possible when you'd walked on a *Sphagnum* raft over a quaking bog. It felt natural to stand beside Susan and Colin on the shores of Llyn-dhu, the Black Lake, where Grimnir the hooded went to live beneath the waters like 'Grendel of old'. And when the children realised the Black Lake lay within Lindow Common, its name derived from the Welsh for black lake, *llyn-dhu*, we were back on familiar ground. Less than a mile away from the real-life Black Lake is Lindow Moss, where, 24 years after the publication of *The Weirdstone of Brisingamen*, Lindow Man rose from the peat.

Between the ages of 11 and 14, my somewhat erratic diary (prefaced with gentle warnings – 'Shoo/Hands Off' – and more truculent admonitions – 'Piss Off/Get Lost!') suggests life revolved around food, music and books. When I wasn't eating or practising, I was reading the next library book, and vice versa. I read as I walked to school, in the playground and under the covers by torchlight, inhabiting the increasingly porous boundary between reality and imagination. I had a wide circle of fictional friends with whom I spent more time than anyone in real life. These one-sided, predictable relationships (safer on every rereading) offered the same kind of security as life in the garden.

The day after my thirteenth birthday, I addressed my diary rather pompously: 'I think I will now tell you something of my life. I was born in the Midlands and here I lived for seven years. Of this time in my life, I do not remember much.' Thinking back to the bombweed years is a curious experience, like weighing a heavy absence I've always felt I carried. I might think it was all a delusion, that I began life in Cheshire, newborn at seven and a half, were it not for the photos.

A sombre little presence, I appear in lots of old slides, often looking pensive or bemused, as if having a camera pointed at me is rather a shock. In one photo where I have a yellow plastic boater balanced on my head, I look downright furious. But every picture taken outdoors shows my big beaming smile. I smile running on the beach, smile as I roll down a grassy hill, orange dress up around my ears, white knickers on display. I smile on a path beside allotments, holding a yellow bucket with my left hand, my Aunty Pauline's hand with my right. I'm positively beaming, sat in the snow in my red all-in-one with go-faster arm stripes. There was clearly a lot of fun to be had outside.

If these early photographs confirm my presence, a sort of *Back to the Future* dissolution kicks in later. I refuse to face the camera, turning away as the shutter comes down. I disappear behind taller photographees or slip round the back before the shot is taken. Still do, given half a chance. I'd always assumed it was self-consciousness about my front teeth after an orthodontist countered my 12-year-old refusal to wear braces because they would alter my flautist's embouchure with the jaw-dropping: "Don't you want to be pretty? Do you really want to look like that for the rest of your life?"

"I'm fine the way I am," I told him, while Mum applauded me silently from the back of the room, but I never forgot his question and its implications. They continued to nibble away at my self-confidence for the next 30 years. But I think there was more to my unwillingness to appear on camera than simply my looks. It was a desire to escape unrecorded, to avoid the visual statement 'I am here'. If you left no trace, no one could pin you down or judge you.

I'm told I was exceedingly reluctant to move away from Nuneaton at the age of seven. On my first morning at my new junior school in Cheshire, I stood in the corner of the classroom, arms outstretched, and declared: "I don't want to be here, but Mummy says I have to come, so don't talk to me." I can believe it. Even now, as I write the words, I feel an unaccountable urge to push my hands towards you, palms out. I'm seven and I'm keeping you at arm's length. Change and me, new people, new situations – we've never been the best of friends. The thought of being the centre of attention, plonked into a classroom of new faces, the curiosity, the stares. Urgh, the stuff of anxious dreams. But having said my piece, it seems I settled in well enough and caused no trouble.

At the end of my first diary entry as a brand-new teenager, I considered my position at secondary school: 'I am fairly happy here. I love the lessons. I am not a particularly sociable person, so I get along on my own at school.' Clearly my people skills had not improved much between the ages of seven and 13. 'I love writing, English, French, German and history. I detest maths. When I am older, I will be an actress, an orchestral flute player, a translator or a writer.' Well, at least I got something right.

When I was ten, I joined the village drama group and discovered another doorway into the world of the imagination. My first pantomime was *Humpty Dumpty* and I was immensely proud of my inaugural role as Humpty Dumpty's understudy. Unfortunately for me, the child playing Humpty was disgustingly healthy, so I had no chance to sit on, or indeed fall off, the wall. But I learned all the words – mine and everyone else's – and it was an honour I never forgot.

My favourite thing about pantomime was the music. Every script came with gaps for musical numbers but no set score.

Instead, our director added songs from a wide range of musicals, operas, films and, my favourites, Gilbert and Sullivan operettas. Mum sometimes played the tinny church hall piano for rehearsals and shows, and she'd practise at home so the music was part of our lives for months. I'd sing panto songs endlessly from September until our production run in March, probably driving the rest of my family to distraction, then enter a period of deep mourning once the show was over.

I loved singing and acting, revelled in the sheer exhilaration of this world of enchantment. Friends and family who knew a little of my reticence to speak in public would sometimes ask me "How come you're so confident on stage?" I wasn't ever sure what to say. When I stepped out of the wings something shifted in my head, that was all. I wasn't me anymore – no longer just a part of other people's lives, a character in their stories. In these imaginary worlds, as I inhabited each new persona, I had a story of my own to tell. On stage, for just a few moments each year, I felt I'd earned the right to be noticed.

I was a dab hand at principal boys and villains (Jack in *The Grand Old Duke of York*, the Prince in *Aladdin*, Chief Weasel in *The Wind in the Willows*), so I was nonplussed and gratified as a 16-year-old to be cast as Princess Talida in *Sinbad the Sailor*. Out with the animal costumes, trousers and bob-cuts; in with grass skirts, skimpy sequinned tops and gazing dreamily into Sinbad's eyes. Normal service resumed, however, the following spring with *The Wizard of Oz*. I'd played a Munchkin in my first year at school, plastered with blue poster paint that cracked and flaked when I smiled. Now, at 17, I landed the Scarecrow: a dream role with comic songs, loose-limbed dancing and lots of slapstick stunts. It was my last panto before leaving for university, my last main part before I lost confidence and sought anonymity in the chorus line. Playing the Scarecrow, singing 'If I Only Had a Brain' and dancing like a fool on that much-loved stage was the highlight of my childhood.

I inherited my love of music from my mum. By the time I was five, Mum had started giving piano lessons from home. She taught me for a few years before I moved on to another teacher, and I have vague recollections of sitting next to her on the piano stool, learning scales and arpeggios. I never wanted to be a soloist, but I enjoyed accompanying people and playing show tunes. I still love playing the piano today.

I recall the feeling of bubbling excitement when Mum and I boarded coaches on dark winter evenings to travel to the ballet or opera in Liverpool or Manchester. My amazement at the tiny red opera glasses, so ineffectual compared to the big binoculars my dad used to look at birds, and plush auditoriums where you left your empty ice cream tubs under your seats – "Really, Mum, are we actually allowed to do that?" Outside the auditorium, Mum passed on her love of Gilbert and Sullivan through the tapes we sang along to in the car. And every summer in the late 1980s, we'd meet up with my uncle, aunt and cousins at Gawsworth Hall, just down the road from their house, to see G & S operettas performed by a stellar cast including several members of the D'Oyly Carte Opera Company. I adored these open-air productions – *Patience, Iolanthe, The Mikado, Yeoman of the Guard* – and our family picnics in the gardens beforehand. The second act took place as long summer evenings faded to dusk, and afterwards we walked back through the grounds in the dark. Our yearly G & S trips in July signalled the beginning of my summer.

These recollections of Mum and music have been folded away in the back of my mind for so long that almost all their detail has been lost in the creases. When I open out the years, any surviving memories of my mum are as fragile as paper snowflakes. The tears that her illness rent in our relationship nearly a half-century ago, once unfolded, unleash a snowstorm of perforations. Among the little that remains is the sound of an orchestra awakening as its notes meet the fresh evening air, the heady perfume and velvet skin of the Opera House, and the tomtit singing "Willow, tit willow, tit willow."

When I was seven, I told my parents that I wanted to play the flute. I rarely asked for anything, so they agreed and bought me a Boosey & Hawkes silver flute in a blue leather case. I knew from the outset it was the only solo instrument for me. The rich sweetness of the notes beguiled me; playing felt like a physical expression of the beauty of music. Alongside playing the flute and piano, I joined the school choir, learning to use my singing voice confidently in public in a way I could not match in speech. By the time I moved to secondary school, music was an integral part of my life.

When I was 13, I came across Antonio Salieri (1750–1825), a composer, conductor and music teacher. Salieri was Wolfgang Amadeus Mozart's arch-rival, a watcher in the shadows if you believe Peter Shaffer's depiction of him as a schemer in his 1979 play *Amadeus*, later adapted into the 1984 film of the same name. I'd advise against unquestioning acceptance of this fictionalised portrayal of Salieri, but as a mardy teen watching the film at my cousin Arwen's house (sleeping at night on the piano room floor, attending singing courses every day in the foothills of the Pennines), I swallow the story whole. *I am Salieri*, I think. Paean to mediocrity. Like him, I will observe and teach. Like him, I'll appreciate genius and follow in its wake.

Salieri both adored and despised Mozart's musicality, having failed to compose pieces that ascended to the same celestial heights himself. Like millions of others, no doubt, I have played and sung Mozart's music throughout my life, but not Salieri's. Listening to Mozart's *Exsultate, Jubilate* a few years ago in St Mary's Church in Hitchin, I was transported nearly 40 years into the past, to another St Mary's, this time in Conwy, North Wales, where I waited in the shadows for my own solo as part of the lunchtime concert series. I was nine and about to play one of my favourite pieces, possibly Mozart's 'Andante in C' or 'To A Wild Rose' by American composer Edward MacDowell. I remember being scared, even in the modest church with its sparse audience, but once the accompaniment began, I knew I'd be at peace.

Psallant aethera cum me
(Let the heavens sing forth with me)
It is always shadow-rimmed
And stone cold in that church
But music brings me light.

Exsultate, Jubilate
In liquid fire from a lone soprano
Cascading down the nave
Pouring over pews

Bathing the congregation
In rejoicing.

> *My heart sighs with yours*
> *Stirring forgotten motes, composing memories*
> *In response to your singing.*

Salieri-like, against a damply crusted pillar
Half stone, half dust
I listen (aspiring,

My nine-year-old fingers poised
For communion with each padded key
For the anticipated immersion in silversonic peace).

> *My heart sighs with yours*
> *Stirring forgotten motes, composing memories*
> *In response to your singing.*

Centuries later, I emerge into salty dazzle
Fresh and alive, noteworthy
With Alleluias playing in my soul.

I loved playing for other people, but hated the waiting and those first few seconds in the spotlight before the performance began. How did Stephen do it, I wonder? My younger brother, facing the congregation in Manchester Cathedral week after week, just visible across the nave in a line of ethereal little boy faces. I'm not sure I'd have had the courage to fill that space, to soar with those treble voices. Or travel into Manchester every day to music school and most weekends too – a tiring two-hour round trip for a ten-year-old. Not that I was given the opportunity. My voice would have been considered inferior, lacking the 'purity' of a boy's treble. I was allowed to listen, but not to sing. Manchester Cathedral Choir had no spaces for girls.

Perhaps Stephen felt scared too, when he began. If so, it didn't stop him. He sang with Manchester Cathedral Choir from the age of 11 to 13, and at 19 won a choral scholarship to Trinity College, Cambridge. The Choir of Trinity College was ahead of its time – female students had been admitted from 1982 – but not all colleges were, or indeed are, so inclusive. King's College Choir still accepts only male students and choristers, although there is also a mixed college choir called King's Voices. The college website explains that becoming a chorister at King's is 'probably the best musical education available to children between the ages of 9 and 13', then goes on to say they're looking for boys with a love of music and singing. Even in the twenty-first century, old traditions die hard.

In Durham Cathedral, where I sang with the University Choral Society for ten years while studying and working in the city, there's a line of local black Frosterley marble across the floor at the west end of the nave. It marks a boundary over which women were not allowed to pass. Fortunately, that was a few years before my time. By the mid-sixteenth century, this marker of female exclusion was merely a decorative feature and women had access to the whole nave. It would, however, be another 450 years before the cathedral opened its choir stalls to girls, in 2009.

In 1995, when I was 20, Manchester Cathedral finally welcomed girls as choristers. It was one of the first cathedrals to do so

– an early pioneer in terms of gender equality – but a decade too late for me. I'm not bitter. If music was a schoolgirl crush (choirs, musicals, orchestral concerts, three hours of flute practice a day to achieve Grade 8 distinction – my passport to the Young Musician of the Year, I hoped, though I bottled it before applying), then writing became my soulmate from my late teens onwards. I don't regret swapping notes for letters, chords for words. But I am glad that times have changed. I couldn't become a chorister, but my daughter can join a cathedral choir if she wishes. She could audition to sing in nearby St Albans Cathedral Girls Choir, formed in 1996 (the boys' choir is still referred to as the St Albans Cathedral Choir). In fact, she prefers to dance and practise acrobatic arts, but at least she has the choice. Unless she wants to sing in the Choir of Westminster Abbey, of course. Then she'd still have to be a boy.

Despite my Salieri-like affinity for lingering in the shadows, I was aware that some of my behaviour in my mid-teens marked me out as an attention-seeker. Though a generally cheerful and compliant kid, I became increasingly introverted at school, withdrawing completely in some lessons, incapable of taking part in discussions or speaking assessments. I'd write, words flowed with ease on the page but they faltered in my throat and dried up before they left my lips. I became a shadow-child in class, trying to efface myself so I wouldn't be noticed or called upon to speak. Although I was trying to disappear, ironically my behaviour called attention to myself, and I sensed this. I was aware on some level that it was a cry for help and I hated myself for it. It felt like the kind of play-acting my mother had been accused of. And I knew I was capable of speaking in other situations – at home, on stage – so assumed (following my teachers' lead) that my confusing inability to talk in class was wilful defiance. But I'm starting to realise this behaviour was an instinctive stress response rather than an intentional ploy, and I can see how it has matured into the dissociation and social anxiety that still makes life hard today. We talk about 'losing sight of' or 'losing touch with' – I lost sound of my own voice. And, trapped in silence, I lost faith in my own integrity. I knew women exaggerated and falsified, so I repressed difficult feelings. I had no right to strong emotions.

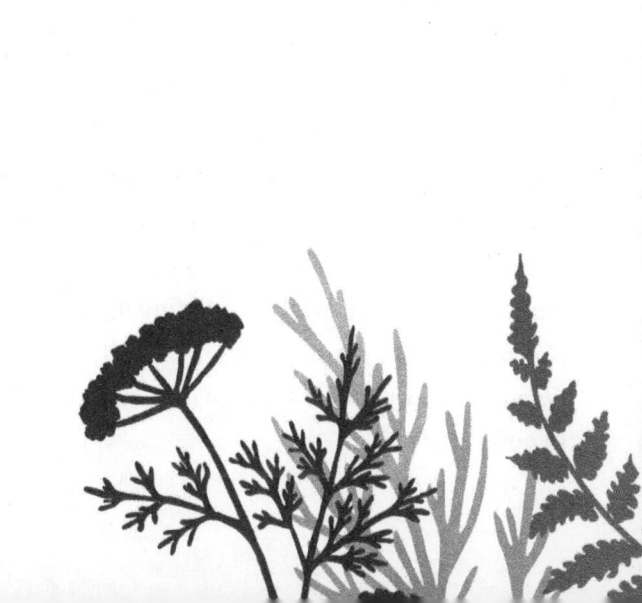

I've had this recurring dream since I was a kid. I'm standing in the entrance hall of our old bungalow facing the dark-green rotary dial phone. I'm frightened. I don't like using it and I push my index finger into the stiff coils of cord as far as it will go. They tighten and hold me. But I need to make a call, so I pull it back out and start to dial. My fingertip slides in the number hole. I drag the dial round and hear the long whirr and click as it unwinds. Even though I know the number, every time I get near the end I misdial and have to start again. The digits swim in front of me, swapping places like the consonants do when I'm trying to pronounce long words. Panic rises. I'll never be able to talk. I'm on my own and I need help.

This dream stalked me into adulthood, long after rotary dial phones were just a retro memory. My subconscious kept up to date though, downloading the latest technology so now I had to make the call on a push-button phone. An easier task, you'd think, in an emergency. Not so. My finger still struggled to find the right buttons. It was always the last numbers that got in a muddle. I'd be nearly there, the beginnings of relief, then a mistouch and I'd have to start all over again. Now mobile phones have simplified the communication process even further. No need to punch in a string of numbers at all. Phone on – Unlock – Contacts – Select ICE. I can ring my 'In Case of Emergency' contact with four screen clicks.

But I had the dream again last week. I'm cold and scared. This time I'm trapped in a cable car halfway down a cliff and I need to speak to someone, to call for help. But I can't work my mobile. Or perhaps it's not mine. I don't recognise the operating system and, no matter which way I swipe, I can't find my numbers. No apps screen. No contacts list. No ICE. I know there's help available. It's just a phone call away. But it's been over 30 years and I've never managed to make that call.

The Wood Between the Worlds

It's 1.29 p.m., 9 September 2021. My first session is about to begin. I press the 'join meeting' button and my counsellor appears in a box next to me on-screen. She has a mournful, piecemeal face made up from bits of other people's stories. I only see it for a moment, then she asks me why I've come for counselling and I can't make eye contact anymore. I can't speak either and it's no longer me in the room. I'm watching the scene from far away: two women side by side on-screen and a third at the desk. Time passes so slowly – a pause that stretches until it is no longer plausible that the woman at the desk is simply gathering her thoughts. There are no thoughts. I've misplaced myself, withdrawn to a muted hinterland like C. S. Lewis's Wood Between the Worlds, where life is suspended and memories drift through the trees. I'm familiar with this green sanctuary (I've been here many times before), but I'm an adult now and I know there's somewhere else I ought to be.

There are many ways out of the wood, and the path I follow leads not to my study, but to the top floor of the English block in my comprehensive school, to a moment I thought I'd forgotten years ago. But here I am again, frozen in an eternity of panic, staring mutely at my desk. The lesson has ended but I'm not allowed to leave, because I have to explain to my English teacher why I don't speak in class. The impossibility of his demand seems obvious to me, but he doesn't get it. He is tall and his stomach leans towards me over his belt. He reeks of exasperation and aftershave. He outranks me physically in every way, but he thinks 'arid' means fertile and he likes to make his students debate corporal punishment and the benefits of the death penalty. Up here the classroom is all windows and light, but the smell of aftershave is making me queasy and I feel like I might fall. He wants to know why I won't answer questions or participate in lessons. I don't remember his exact words, but they're asking for information I don't have and anyway I can't reply, so there's no conversation to recall.

I wonder if he knows I have form in this department. I hope no one's told him about the English lessons last term when I sat, head buried in my arms on the desk, trying to ignore the numbness inside and the excruciatingly slow class reading of *Hobson's Choice* going on around me. I remember getting a right bollocking one afternoon for being purposely sullen and difficult. I guess I deserved it, but I felt confused at the same time. Why couldn't I look up in lessons? Why wouldn't my voice work? What was wrong with me? My teacher gave up on me in the end. She stopped asking me to read aloud or answer questions. It felt like I didn't exist anymore and I wasn't sure if I'd won or lost.

Now in my fourth year, this loathing of English lessons has solidified into a cold dread. My stomach turns every time I enter the classroom and my anxiety grows as the months pass. We are expected to have strong opinions and talk about our emotions.

But I've had a lot of practice at keeping my emotions to myself. I can't always find them, let alone parade them in front of other people who respond in confusing and unpredictable ways. And it doesn't help that I'm tactless. I know I am because Mum told me so and I know she considers it a bad trait. I wrote it in my school report in my first and second year, on the list of Things to Improve: 'Be more tackful'. I can spell it now, but I still don't know how to do it, because Mum never explained how I lost my tact in the first place or where I might find it again. I also know I'm selfish and manipulative and have things called 'ulterior motives'. I struggle to find them but I do search about in my head sometimes, rummaging round like I'm after a lost biro at the bottom of my school bag. I don't doubt they're in there somewhere. Adults know these things. I don't though, so it seems safer to keep my opinions to myself.

None of this helps me explain to my English teacher why I keep failing my GCSE speaking tests. I remain frozen without answers, staring at the desk in the top floor classroom. There's no resolution, so I can't work through the memory and lay it to rest. The only escape is through the wood and back to my study. I feel a little more present now I've returned. I sit up straighter in my chair and look my counsellor in the eye and her face looks kind and whole and I can see she is waiting for me to tell her my story.

By the end of the session, I'd managed to say a few words, though it would be weeks before I could answer her questions fully. My sudden physical inability to move or respond when my counsellor spoke to me reminds me how distressing I found it when anxiety and stress triggered similar dissociative episodes at school. I think I got some kind of special dispensation for my inability to talk in speaking tests in the end. I imagine it would have been rather embarrassing if a straight-A student had failed GCSE English. But I don't remember anyone asking me why it was happening. And even if they had, I'd been given no words to describe the situation at home, no way to express the sense of underlying sadness and anxiety that I couldn't even recognise myself. Who was I to feel anything when Mum was feeling so much? And if her illness wasn't acknowledged by the mainstream medical profession and we were given no framework or compassionate terminology with which to discuss it, what chance did we have to understand her suffering and its effect on us as a family? It wasn't until decades later I could look back past my self-loathing to that sometimes-mute, attention-seeking child and recognise my own pain.

I worked hard in my late teens to overcome my difficulties speaking in class. My sixth form report confirms my developing ability to contribute, though it also mentions perfectionism and a tendency to be over-anxious. In biology lessons I was, apparently, 'a great worrier'. My English teacher describes me as 'exciting and stimulating to work with', but notes I was 'almost too highly motivated'. Her advice was to stop worrying about my abilities – just relax and enjoy it.

Unlike most of my friends, I split my subject choices across the arts/sciences divide. I took English, French, biology and maths (I discovered a love of numbers once it became more challenging).

In terms of careers, I vacillated between marine biology and English teaching. My interest in aquatic life began in the watery depths of my form room at secondary school. My tutor was a biology teacher, so every morning we'd pull our lab stools up to the old lacquered benches, pitted and scored by generations of wood-boring students. Fish tanks lined the walls. Long strings of bubbles rose intermittently and pond snails studded the greenish glass. In the chemistry lab next door, I'd sit at my desk during lessons staring out of the long science block windows onto the playground below, but in my form room I could lose myself in a subaquatic world. My form tutor was a keen diver and angler, so he'd teach us about fish and other freshwater and marine creatures. He was quick to laugh, slow to anger, and he looked out for me for years. Some mornings, when life at home was tough, he'd come in and give me a wink. It meant 'Are you okay? I'm here if you need me.' In my underwater form room, I felt safe and seen.

During my GCSE biology field trip to the Menai Strait – the thin strip of sea separating the Isle of Anglesey from Gwynedd on the Welsh mainland – I learned more about marine ecology. Our transect studies in the intertidal zone encouraged close-up encounters with seaweed, sea snails, crabs, sandhoppers and a whole host of creatures that thrived in this fluid environment. I still remember the Latin name for bladderwrack – *Fucus vesiculosus* – a mysterious incantation that I repeated to myself throughout the week like a marine mantra, and how my form teacher showed us the groove in the dog whelk's shell through which the sea snail extends a siphon for respiration and to detect the scent of its mussel and barnacle prey. Those summer days exploring rock pools and seaweed-strewn tidelines felt like a rerun of holidays when I was a little kid staying with my grandparents in Conwy. I enjoyed the field trip so much that I went along again, as a student helper, the summer after I left school.

But when my A level course moved from ecology to cell and human biology, I was less than enthusiastic. I felt we'd already learned more than enough about the disturbing female body at GCSE. I was still haunted by the chart where potential complications of pregnancy were helpfully laid out for us: gestational diabetes, high blood pressure, pre-eclampsia, depression; the list went on and on, before we even reached giving birth. I read it with mounting disbelief. Why would anyone put themselves through that? Why invite illness in if you were well? Pregnancy was clearly a mug's game. Whereas natural history seemed scientific and objective, human biology felt uncomfortably close to home. I wanted to look outwards not inwards, so I dropped the course at the end of my lower sixth.

With English literature now my main focus, I joined the Oxbridge study group and set my sights on a place at St Catharine's College, Cambridge. The legendary university seemed to me, at 17, the pinnacle of all ambition. I loved the extra tuition and spread my literary wings with personal recommendations from my teacher. I was captivated by prose – *Under the Volcano* by Malcolm Lowry, *Chatterton* by Peter Ackroyd, John Fowles's *The Magus,* the all-consuming worlds of A. S. Byatt's *Possession* and Salman Rushdie's *Midnight's Children*. I devoured every D. H. Lawrence, Thomas Hardy and E. M. Forster novel I could get my hands on, and read the Cambridge literary critics – F. R. Leavis, I. A. Richards and William Empson, never once wondering why I was being weaned on such a male diet. We practised interviews and, little by little, I became more confident talking about myself and my insatiable appetite for literature.

On the day of the interview, we followed the motorway signs to 'The SOUTH' to an arcane city I'd read about only in books and a university I'd not have been surprised to find a mirage of my literary imagination. My memories of the interview are hazy; I was overawed by the grandeur of the colleges, the effervescent confidence of the other candidates. So far out of my comfort zone I almost forgot who and what I was. When the interviewer asked about authors I enjoyed – the most undemanding of all questions – every book I'd ever read just melted away. Primal biology kicked in. The familiar sensation of shutdown in progress. Panic and embarrassment at the nakedness of my mind.

Years later, I'd talk through this process with A level students in the study skills department of the sixth form college where I worked. Students were often referred to me because they struggled with exam stress or essay writing. I remembered exactly how it felt to lose access to knowledge you'd worked hard to retain. I'd explain it was perfectly natural. When under stress, the areas of the brain responsible for executive functions, such as working memory, can shut down as the limbic system – the part responsible for the fight, flight or freeze reaction – takes over. "Don't worry," I'd tell my students, "the information hasn't gone for good. Practice and relaxation techniques can help you manage this stress response."

I wish someone had explained it like that to me. Given me a reason why my brain (and body) would sometimes suddenly, sullenly seize up. Told me it was an entirely natural biological process and not a personal flaw. Instead, when I received my rejection from St Catharine's, it confirmed what I'd always suspected. I wasn't good enough. I'd fancied myself better than I was and, like the tragic heroes I was studying, I'd had my comeuppance.

The next few weeks passed in a fug of depression. I cried my way through the sixth form days and lost nearly a stone in weight from the scanty starting point of seven and a half stone. Academic success had always been fundamental to my sense of identity; it was how I proved my worth and, up to this point, hard graft had enabled me to achieve anything I set my mind to. Now I'd reached my limits and I was completely devastated. It seems ridiculous, looking back, to have been so affected by what I suspect was the luckiest failure of my life. If friends' experiences are anything to go by, the intensity of life in Cambridge would likely have exacerbated my own tendencies towards anxiety and perfectionism. But, at the time, it felt like the end of the world.

Soon afterwards I grudgingly agreed to visit Durham for my final university interview. I fell in love with the city the moment the train crossed the viaduct south of the station and I saw the 900-year-old cathedral rising from a peninsula formed by the River Wear. Without the esoteric associations of Cambridge and, after a couple of days staying in college (a requirement for all interviewees), I was already finding my feet in this quirky, friendly city. I knew the college had an excellent reputation for student support – a team I was privileged to join when I became a pastoral tutor after graduating – and a few weeks after my interview I accepted a place at Durham. Over the next three years, my brother and cousins all gained places at Cambridge and moved down south. I upped sticks too, heading around the Yorkshire Dales and across the North Pennines to start a new life in the North East.

I was a peripatetic hill-dweller during my decade in Durham, living high on each side of the city except the north. As well as staying in college on Elvet Hill just off South Road, I shared a weed-ridden house with three lads on a hill in the east, in part of what was once a mining area. In later years, my boyfriend and I rented a semi at the top of Western Hill. Only one year passed on flat ground, in a three-storey building called Kepier Lodge down by the River Wear. It was the grandest place I'd ever lived – a lucky find through a landlord friend. Once part of the Kepier Hospital estate established around 1180, the area had included a church, tannery, bakery, mill and farm with large orchard and, in later years, a Victorian penitentiary for so-called fallen women surrounded by a wall studded with broken glass. As the only woman sharing a house with seven men ("One for every day of the week..." I'd quip if friends raised their eyebrows at me), I managed to wangle the top spot – a vast airy chamber on the second floor with bookcases spanning one entire wall. My own private reading room.

Standing at the elevated sash window, I could look out over the River Wear and a large area of grassland along the riverbank called The Sands. Sometimes I'd see goosanders diving for fish, the drakes slick-splendid with those iridescent green heads, and wicked sawbills. These days I love to watch females (the redheads) too, but when I first spotted goosanders on the river, I only had eyes for the males. In the spring, swallows and sand martins would appear, swooping low over the water before disappearing up and over Milburngate Bridge in the direction of the cathedral. But it's not just the birds I remember. Walking into the city early one morning, I looked up along The Sands. Two camels were approaching. I did a double take. They were still approaching. And it wasn't as if anything I'd drunk the previous evening should have caused Bactrian hallucinations. The Freemen of Durham had ancient herbage rights to graze cows, sheep, goats and horses on this common land – though I'd only ever seen dogs chasing balls across the grass – but camels? Then up ahead: trailers, tents, a few folk milling around. The circus had come to town. Every time I looked out of my window for the next few days, I'd see the unlikely duo roaming The Sands, feasting on leathery lipfuls of fresh grass.

My happiest Durham memories are those of my three years living in college. Almost all my friends were guys, mostly maths, physics and computing students. We were a pretty chilled-out set. Hanging around in our shared rooms; chasing adventure in the fantasy landscapes of Civilization and Myst; listening to music: Alice Cooper, Metallica, Megadeth (one of my boyfriends was a metalhead and a lover of tight faux snakeskin boots), Combustible Edison, They Might Be Giants, Adiemus.

We whiled away our evenings playing Magic: The Gathering or Dungeons & Dragons. Ate cheese and pepperoni toasties, drank QC or Snakebite and Black and chatted past midnight. Or at least, my friends did. "It must be ten o'clock," someone would chime, regular as clockwork, "Nic's fallen asleep again." *She'll sleep anywhere, in anyone's bed.* Our running joke. Next morning I'd wake back in my own room or my boyfriend's, one of the lads having scooped me up in the early hours and carried me home. It never occurred to me to wonder why I zonked out while they all partied on. Why I was neither night owl nor lark. We simply laughed about it. Looking back now, it doesn't seem so funny. It was the beginning of an unravelling, though it was years before I realised the joke was on me.

Fortunately, my studies allowed me plenty of time to read and sleep. My timetable – often no more than one or two lectures a day with the occasional tutorial or seminar thrown in for good measure – was a source of amusement, and not a little irritation, to my scientist friends with their jam-packed schedules. The blue tits would wake me in the morning, long after the others had breakfasted and set off for lectures. Tap-tap-tap. Tap-tap-pop. Cheeky beaks plunged through foil bottle tops to half-inch the cream off the milk I stored on the window ledge.

On Sunday mornings I'd lie in my boyfriend's bed listening to Classic FM Romance, watching rabbits plucking daisies on the lawn, noses twitching, nibbling up the stems until they sported a faceful of flower. Sometimes, after too long penned in with Chaucer or the metaphysical poets, I'd nip across the road and wander under the beeches in Great High Wood, or idle round the Botanic Garden enjoying the planting, doubling back with my boyfriend after hours to find a leafy spot for some decidedly non-botanical activities. Life was free and easy. Sorted.

This is how I remember my university years. Love, laughter and good company in a city I adored with all my heart. A genial tale I've told myself; all of it true. An idyllic period when I outgrew my childhood anxieties. But I'd buried too much, too deep and it was biding its time. Though I felt bolder and wiser, more myself than I'd ever been, I hadn't yet figured out how to talk about my feelings. My instinctive response to overwhelming stress was still to retreat inside my own head, and soon it began to cause dissociative shutdown far more extreme than anything I'd experienced before.

As always, it started with denial. The suppression of difficult emotions I had no right to experience or express...

"Don't make a fuss."
"Pull yourself together."
"Don't be so dramatic."

Imperatives from another time, another life. Old voices in my head. But I'm done with obedience. Sometimes you have to take yourself apart, lay out the drama of the past and work through the fuss you didn't make before you can pull yourself back together again.

Early hours of a cold March morning. Flappers and dandies partying hard after our final performance of the roaring twenties musical *The Boy Friend*: an apt show for a time when I broke up with my own boyfriend and found a new one, though not necessarily in that order. The dancing was intense; my head was spinning. Not from the effects of alcohol, as I didn't drink (too much danger of uncontrolled emotion there). Instead, I was swept up in a whirlwind of exhaustion and an increasing sense of guilt. I'd fallen for suave playboy Bobby Van Husen in our very first rehearsal – that beautiful singing voice, his sense of humour, his dancing – but couldn't find the words to end my current relationship.

Music pulsed, our bodies hot and close, my emotions rising. I pushed them down as always, but this time the old approach failed me. Pulsing, dancing, pressing, my body, my head, eyes shut tight, walls closing, trapped inside, no way out. Deep I went, so deep the music faded and the dancing ceased. Inside my head I finally ran out of places to hide. No way to retreat any further or make myself any smaller.

On the outside, my body went rigid, then the convulsions began. I remember the vague sensation of being lifted and carried off the dance floor; hearing a siren from a distance as if it were the soundtrack to someone else's story; coming round in the ambulance on the way to hospital; trying to swallow horribly sweet tea as I sat on the bed in A & E, dazed and frightened. I remember my indignant response to the inevitable question. Of course I hadn't been taking drugs. I hadn't needed to. My body had provided the adrenaline to fuel my internal escape.

Sitting here on my narrow windowsill, writing about my seizure, I'm hyperaware of the tension in my calves, thighs, forearms, upper arms and shoulders, the drop to my right, how precarious it would be to lose myself right now. Recalling that first seizure awakens these muscle memories. Recalling the second relies on borrowed memories. Details of the past returned to me by the boyfriend who observed and remembered what I dismissed and forgot.

I was at a garden party. A large gathering of my new boyfriend's family and friends, most of whom had known each other for years. As a shy introvert, this was far from my natural environment. I had to talk to people I didn't know: strangers who might judge me. I felt newly visible and somehow guilty, a usurper taking the place of a well-liked ex-girlfriend, who was also at the party. I tried to mingle and attempted light conversation. I think there were apple trees at the bottom of the garden. Possibly it was a sunny afternoon. Certainly, there was food – at a time when coeliac disease had not yet marked me as an outsider.

At some point I felt anxiety churning in the pit of my stomach, prompting the physical need to escape, yet I was bounded by the knowledge that to do so would forever label me as *that* girlfriend, the one who did an antisocial runner at the summer party. Perhaps I told myself to stand firm, to breathe deep down and focus. But I'd found a way out now and I guess it wasn't long before muscle memory took over.

Physically   Mentally

                tensing   retracting

        becoming rigid   a snail-shelled

                juddering   safety

Was I protected inside that hard convulsive casing? For a while, at least. But the emotions were still there, waiting for me on my return.

The third, fourth, fifth seizures... and the rest? Those I remember. How could I forget? Always the same triggers. Guilt. Pleasure. Guilty pleasure. Though why it felt guilty I couldn't say. Perhaps for the same reason that laying it out now feels at once liberating and humiliating. It's a story I want to tell and it is mine to tell, though I'm sure it's not mine alone. But somewhere inside my head a scolding voice warns me to keep my personal life to myself. Nice girls do not wash their dirty linen in public.

Screw that, I think, moving backwards to ferret through feelings I need to examine and understand. Onwards too, to the woman

I want to become. But I can't stop my muscles tensing and shuddering as if someone has just opened the October windows beside me and let in a raw blast of air.

I look out at the ash tree across the street and force myself to face memories I've tried – and failed – to forget. Something that happened so often it began to feel inevitable. Pleasure then pain. Sex then seizure. *La petite mort* resurrected in the convulsions of a full-blown fit. In the midst of my distress, I was aware of a body struggling on the bed, but it wasn't mine. How could it be when I was so far away, protected from the backlash, just a foetal curl inside my own head?

Watching me have a seizure must have been a disturbing experience for my partner. But I managed not to end up in an ambulance again, and I never went to the doctor. I was too scared, too ashamed of my loss of control and the circumstances surrounding it. So I didn't find out what was causing the seizures, not until many years later. Instead, I followed my usual strategy. I ignored them. And, in time, their severity decreased. Eventually they stopped altogether. I even started to talk a bit when I felt guilty or frightened. But the best way for me to deal with difficult emotions has always been to go outside and give myself space. With the horizon in front and the wind at my back, I can withdraw softly and come to at my own pace in a place where no walls can close around me.

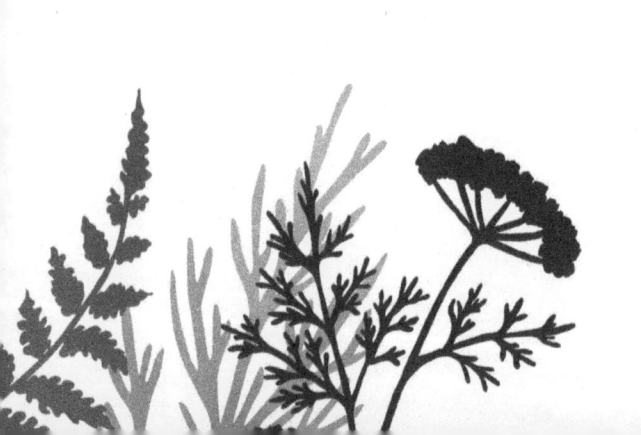

The Road
Less Travelled

I think about walking the Coast to Coast footpath from Cumbria to Robin Hood's Bay, travelling across Europe, helping lead expeditions in the White Mountains in America, going on birding holidays, visiting friends, taking students to the theatre to watch *The Rivals*, *Othello*, *The Crucible* and other plays I was teaching.

I think about these opportunities. All offered to me. All turned down.

I think about 25 years of feeling less than.

I think about how my choices seemed logical at the time, predetermined by living inside an unreliable body.

I think about how I've protected myself from risk and embarrassment.

I think about the way my decisions have tamed me, turned me into someone I don't really recognise or perhaps someone I know only too well but wish I didn't.

I think about the roads I could have taken but chose not to, and wonder who I'd have become had I travelled regardless.

I think I no longer believe in my own body-logic.

I think I will make different decisions in future.

So when did I choose the road less travelled? Perhaps when I was 16, during a trip with my parents and brother from Manitoulin Island in Lake Huron to Kingston on the shores of Lake Ontario...

Our first visit to Canada, five years earlier, had been financed by the inattention of a local millionaire who crashed his brand-new Rolls Royce (3 miles on the clock) into the side of our car as Dad drove us home after a weekend away. The impact broke two of Dad's ribs and wrote off our eight-year-old Renault 14. It left me with a gash behind my ear and a hearty contempt for posh blokes in posh cars. Even though he'd turned without looking, he tried to avoid paying damages, the shameless weasel. He lost in court. We were awarded £2,000 – the price of four plane tickets to Canada. I figured a few bangs and scrapes were fair compensation for a whole summer in a far-off land where I believed the sun always shone. Endless swimming in Lake Ontario and my cousins' pool, fresh sweetcorn straight off the barbecue, the thrill of my first cardinals and hummingbirds.

To an 11-year-old who'd never been anywhere more remote than North Wales before, each new encounter worked like a charm. Eastern garter snakes! Beavers! Snapping turtles! Even the butterflies were bigger. Monarchs swashbuckled through my cousins' garden like flaming stained-glass windows. What were our peacocks or red admirals beside these kings of the butterfly world? As precursors to the orange fire of adulthood, monarch larvae were cool as caterpillars with their zingy yellow, black and white stripes, black tentacles and insouciant taste for toxic plants.

My cousins and I reared them, collecting fresh milkweed from the roadside for our Very Hungry Caterpillars. The long Canadian summer gave us time to follow the stages from larva to pupa to imago – the adult butterfly. I loved watching each winged miracle break through its pupal case and wetly re-enter the world. One day I took one of my monarchs on a lake trip. I knew it was close to hatching as the chrysalis had become transparent and I could see flashes of orange and black, so I piled into the car with my butterfly jar and watched it emerge as we drove along the highway. The newborn monarch enthralled me, hanging there so crumpled and unregal. I watched in awe as its shrunken wings inflated with haemolymph, and I remember my surprise when, all pumped up, it expelled its red meconium right down my shorts.

I have happy memories of our vacations across the pond. Unlike many of our other holidays, where the stress of packing and travelling made Mum ill, she found it relaxing staying with family in Canada. My aunt was a Brownie leader and a whizz at crafts, so Mum and I learned together how to cross-stitch, mould figures out of Fimo modelling clay and make toilet roll people. The highlight of our holidays in Ontario was always the summer picnic at a nearby lake. We'd swim with our cousins, eat hot dogs and ice creams, then enter the races. I remember Toss the Water Balloon, where you had to move increasingly far away from your partner, throwing the balloon without bursting it. We played the same game with raw eggs, with far messier consequences. No matter though, when the lake was right next to us. So easy to clean ourselves with a quick dip. I was hopeless at the tug of war and anything involving sprinting, but my cousin and I won the three-legged race more than once. And our crowning family glory was the year we won the seven-legged race. Most teams of six faltered after a step or two and spent the rest of their time repeatedly falling over beside the start line while the crowd roared with laughter. We gave each set of legs a number and planned a simple chant: "One, two, one, two, one, two". The whistle went and somehow our timing was perfect. We marched towards the finish line without hesitating or stumbling, us younger members of the team practically carried along by the adults. It was a great moment and, like most of our activities in Ontario, a lot of fun.

But during our third holiday in Canada, when I was 16, we set off on an unfortunate road trip. It was the first time we'd ventured so far from my uncle and aunt's home in Kingston and, as we drove back from Manitoulin Island through the Algonquin Provincial Park (with nearly 3,000 square miles of forests and lakes – over three times the size of Cheshire), the sheer scale of Canada's wilderness boggled my English counterpane fields-and-hedgerows mind.

One day we saw black bears – a mother and cub – crossing the road in front of the car. I remember a moose regarding us placidly from the edge of a lake. And where there were lakes, there were loons. Sleek outline, matt-black head, chequerboard back. I thought the great northern diver the most debonair bird I'd ever seen. Its fluid form regards me now from the mantelpiece in the lounge, an aluminium loon on a granite base, a treasured wedding present from my Canadian aunt and uncle. Our wedding invitations are still displayed on our bookcase: two stylised purple divers meeting bill to bill, designed by an artist friend.

Despite bears, moose and loons, the road trip was not a pleasant experience for me. Somewhere along the way I picked up a severe bladder infection. With temperatures exceeding 100 degrees Celsius and long car journeys every day, I guess I became dehydrated and thus more susceptible to bacterial infection. Nothing particularly unusual in this – as many as one in ten girls get a urinary tract infection during childhood, but studies have shown it's more likely in children with active, undiagnosed coeliac disease and that genetic predisposition plays a role in susceptibility. I have a family history of coeliac disease (in my dad's family and likely on my mum's side too) and recurrent UTIs, so perhaps this particular path was predetermined.

Mum and Dad took me to a clinic when we returned to Kingston. The doctors gave me antibiotics to heal my bladder, but couldn't wipe the infection from my mind. I still stung from the acute embarrassment of constantly, urgently needing a wee when the nearest toilets were hours away. Even a few minutes after I'd just been I'd be desperate again and, either as a result of infection or pure anxiety, I couldn't always manage to pee when we reached the restrooms. My uncooperative sphincter muscles would seize up and before I could work out how to relax them again it would be time to head back to the car for more hours of purgatory. I still dream about that seemingly endless drive, still feel the embarrassment rising 30 years later.

Ever since, access to toilets has been an anxious preoccupation for me. Coaches are a no-no, long car journeys so stressful that

I avoid them whenever possible, especially with people I don't know well. Hiking or travelling by minibus with children when I was teaching was also problematic. It's nigh on impossible to slip off quietly to find the conveniences when you're the adult responsible for a large group of students. And my recent diagnosis of adenomyosis suggests another cause for these recurrent problems. Studies have linked the condition to issues of urinary urgency and frequency possibly caused by swelling in the uterus that puts pressure on the bladder too.

Perhaps I might have learned to deal with the worry that I'd need the toilet and rediscovered my travelling confidence in time, had my body not begun to rebel in other ways. Until the end of my teens, energy seemed an infinitely renewable resource. I enjoyed hockey, orienteering and trampolining. Nothing gave me more pleasure than getting out on the water canoeing or windsurfing, except for camping with Guides or Rangers. When I was 13, on my return from Guide Camp with sunburned nose and ears, I confided in my diary that I much preferred to sit and eat on the floor. My greatest desire, right then, was to buy myself a tent so I could live in the garden. Not much has changed, though my preference these days would be for a wood of my own.

I completed my silver Duke of Edinburgh Award with a three-day expedition in the Pennines and got a summer job at a kids' camp in the backwoods of the White Mountain National Forest in New Hampshire. Robert Frost knew this area well. He spent 19 summers in the White Mountains from 1907 onwards, and it was from here in 1912 that he wrote a letter to his friend and editor, Susan Hayes Ward, describing two lonely crossroads he'd walked 'several times this winter' neither of which was 'much traveled'. Perhaps this was the seed-image of his two roads that diverged in a yellow wood – the opening of 'The Road Not Taken', which Frost claimed to be a joke about his friend Edward Thomas's indecisiveness and tendency to regret his choices. In 1915, the year the poem was published in *The Atlantic Monthly*, Frost bought a farm in the town of Franconia. He spent the next five years living here with his family on the western side of the White Mountains.

During my long summer at camp, sandwiched between my second and third years at university, for some unknown reason my body started to leach energy. There never seemed enough evenings or weekends to catch up on all the rest I needed. In retrospect, I think by this time I'd developed coeliac disease: an autoimmune condition that can lie dormant in people who have a specific gene mutation for many years or even your entire life. I don't suppose I'll ever know whether the bladder infection that had caused me so many problems four years earlier activated the disease. It might have been the flu I caught just weeks before I left for America, as several studies suggest some common viral infections could be potential triggers for those who are genetically susceptible. I was laid up for a fortnight. Mum had to lift me up in bed to sip water and, after I recovered, my get-up-and-go had, without question, got up and gone. I made it across the Atlantic – just – but life as a camp counsellor taxed my physical endurance well past its limits. I found it almost impossible to manage the six-day weeks: rising in our shared bunk to Reveille before seven; looking after my group of lively 11-year-olds; working all day; talking or partying after we'd put our young charges to bed. And later, patrolling the grounds on the lookout for skunks (raise the alarm!) and fireflies (enjoy the quiet magic...) until 11 o'clock when our duties ended and I was finally allowed to turn in for the night.

I requested a transfer from campcraft to the music and drama department within the first few days, once I realised how much energy our expeditions demanded and how embarrassing it was to take the kids hiking without easy access to toilets. So I lived and worked all summer of 95 in the White Mountains, just as Frost had done 80 years earlier. I wrote and directed shows, taught the campers musical numbers from *Oliver!*, *Joseph and the Amazing Technicolor Dreamcoat* and *You're a Good Man, Charlie Brown* and accompanied them on the piano. But I didn't take part in the expedition up Mount Washington or lead the kids through the birches on Franconia Notch, the mountain pass the poet could see from his front porch. I'd neither the energy to undertake longer hikes nor the ability to cope without readily available conveniences. When I recall that summer 27 years ago (and perhaps I'm telling this with a sigh), I think Frost's yellow wood was my road not taken.

My camp contract lasted two months but it wasn't long before I was in trouble. However hard I pushed myself, my body couldn't keep going at the same pace and for the same length of time as my fellow counsellors. Unfortunately, my struggles didn't go unnoticed. One day I was called into the principal's office in the vast wooden cabin at the heart of camp and told in no uncertain terms that my attitude wasn't good enough. I must work harder.

Now I have my faults for sure, but I've never been a slacker. I was more used to being advised not to push myself so hard. Being accused of laziness when I felt so close to exhaustion was galling. Soon I began to suffer dizzy spells as well as severe fatigue and I was sent to the medical team, who must have been concerned as they gave me permission to reduce my hours. But with no knowledge of my family history of coeliac disease at this time, no one knew why I was struggling. Over the next few weeks, I think the principal realised I'd been doing as much as my body allowed. When the time came to say goodbye she wished me well, gave me a glowing reference and asked if I would return the following year to write and direct more shows.

I left to travel round America with a friend from camp. We drove to Boston and crossed the continent on the first flight of an economy multi-city package, which involved turning up at an airport and waiting for the next available space on a plane. We spent a few days in a dodgy hostel in San Francisco's red-light district. My only memory of the city is marvelling at the sea lions basking on the docks like giant aquatic slugs. Las Vegas next, to join a tour of both Zion and Bryce Canyon National Park in Utah, stopping on the way to eat watermelons at a homestead in the middle of the desert before driving on to the Grand Canyon.

We stayed with friends from camp in Houston and colleagues from the music department on the outskirts of New York City, in a loft bedroom with a long picture window that looked out over their secluded, tree-lined suburb. Orlando passed in a whirl of rollercoasters, then on to a flea-infested motel in Tampa where alligators lurked in a pond at the bottom of the garden. I ran out of money in this insalubrious establishment and cleaned rooms to pay for my food, but it was worth it for the sunsets and brown pelicans in the bay. At the end of the summer, I flew back across the Atlantic to spend a week with friends in Donegal. I never went back.

I find it hard to believe I made these journeys, over a quarter of a century ago. Now-me is smaller and meeker. Far more risk-averse. She doesn't travel much, certainly not without tedious planning and a backpack full of hard-boiled eggs. But then-me hadn't encountered the comedy of errors that is coeliac disease. My starring role in that gluten-free farce was still many years in the future.

Summer camp was exhausting and nearly broke me, but after three months working and travelling round America, I returned with renewed certainty. I didn't want to spend all of my life in library stacks and lecture theatres. While I loved the desiccated scent and hush of second-hand bookshops, and thrived on the intellectual challenge of writing essays, I also craved fresh air and birds and people. I wanted to study literature, then share my knowledge with young people in the community. I wanted to be a bridge between worlds – a teacher. I discovered I was happiest with my head in a book and my feet firmly on the ground.

I didn't come across environmental writing or psychogeography until many years after my degree, but I was always drawn to writers rooted in landscape and place. In between lectures, I lost myself in the immense pine forests and tremendous precipices of the Apennines in thrall to the Gothic; peered into the depths where Alph, the sacred river, ran through caverns measureless to man; set out to memorise 'The Song of Hiawatha' so I too could learn the language of beasts, their names and all their secrets. I stood with Mariana in the moated grange sighing over the blackest moss, the glooming flats, the flower-plots. My special topic on Eliot and Hardy took me back to Warwickshire, to Mary Ann Evans's birth at South Farm, Arbury, 156 years before I came into the world a mile and a half away in the George Eliot Hospital. I explored Middlemarch, Hayslope and Raveloe; then on to the distant county of Wessex where I visited Casterbridge and roamed Edgon Heath.

My tour guide for many of these fictional journeys was Professor Watson, a truly inspiring lecturer who took us for Eliot, Hardy and the Romantic poets. I went on one of his Lake District reading parties in my second year – a rare opportunity to explore the relationship between poetry and place. During the long weekend, we attended lectures on the influence of landscape on poetry and followed in the Lake Poets' footsteps up Loughrigg Fell and Heron Pike. Dick Watson, who ran these yearly reading parties for a decade, recently sent me photographs of the trip. Most show us on Loughrigg Terrace, looking out towards Grasmere, probably the spot where (according to Dick, whose memory is better than my own) he held forth on the people who had walked there.

Perhaps unsurprisingly, I don't appear on any of the close-ups on the fell. For a moment, I wonder if I was there at all. But then, with the aid of my hand lens, I spy a small figure in one photo descending a series of steps along the fellside and recognise my walking boots (still in the cupboard, though they're relegated to second-best pair now on account of their decrepit seams), my washed-out jeans and blue cagoule. On another, I'm sat at the back of the group at dinner, identifiable by my bob-cut and petite profile.

The final photo – a striking view out of the jaws of Rydal Cave – reminds me of the Salvator Rosa landscapes I used to study with students when I lectured on the Gothic. At first glance you're struck by the chiaroscuro of the shadowy cave-frame stark against the pale clouds. Lean in a little closer and your eye is drawn to the requisite windswept tree spreading athwart the shallow lake – a lone ash still awaiting its spring leaf-cover when we visited just after Easter. In the centre of the image, a line of larches towers over a band of tiny figures. For this one I layer up magnifying glass and hand lens, and there I am, standing next to the professor, who has his hand above his eyes as he peers into the darkness. I wonder what he was saying as we contemplated the old slate mine. Perhaps he was noting the romantic character of the place, straight out of *The Mysteries of Udolpho*. Whatever it was, I remember the awe I felt that weekend when I discovered it was possible, in the right spot with the right knowledge, to transcend the present and exist – untethered – in a landscape of synchronous experiences.

When I graduated, Mum ended up sitting next to Dick at the college dinner. He spoke warmly of me. I was a breath of fresh air in the department, he said. I wonder if his words explained why I always felt a little out of place, like I didn't fit into what seemed, at times, a rather stuffy mould. Perhaps there was a little too much of the scientist, the naturalist, the historian in me? And not everyone appreciates undergraduates who stir up the dust as they pass through.

Some of my lecturers – one in particular to whom I awarded 'human being points' if I observed any empirical evidence during tutorials that he existed in the real world – were dismissive of pluralists like me; their idea of the intellectual apogee was that of the specialist (preferably poetry) critic or literary theorist in rarefied fields like postmodernism or poststructuralism, which seemed so far removed from reality that I rechristened them 'hyperbolic studies'. My love of the novel and fascination with the interplay between disciplines was seen by some as evidence of a second-class mind. When I began my dissertation on Jungian psychology in *The Lord of the Rings*, I was told outright that not everyone would see J. R. R. Tolkien as worthy of university study. In the end it was marked by a lecturer who included fantasy among his specialisms. He gave it a first.

Fortunately, he wasn't the only one who sympathised with my less than canonical interests. I'd often bump into my favourite tutor, the late Professor Michael O'Neill (at the time a lecturer younger than I am now), in the gym. As well as being a world-renowned authority on Romanticism, he was a gifted teacher, a poet and a thoroughly lovely man. When he died far too young in 2018, student tributes poured in. They included one from a fresher he'd found lost outside his office in her first week (he sat her down to work out her entire term's timetable with her) and another from a student who described him as the first lecturer to give him the go-ahead for his dissertation on comics.

Michael encouraged my interest in fantasy. At the end of one tutorial, he gave me a critical study of C. S. Lewis, which I still have, its pages warped and swollen after he dropped it in the bath some 25 years ago. It was rather a surprise (and good to know) that some lecturers were real people who read – albeit clumsily – in the bath. Even now I struggle to view academics and authors, including those whom I count as friends, as real people rather than part of some imaginary coterie. My inability to rid myself of this early idealism fuels my imposter syndrome. How can I be a writer when I doubt myself and make so many mistakes, when I spend hours hanging up the socks and loading the dishwasher, when I am so undeniably ordinary? Clearly this is nonsense, yet the fiction persists.

In the third year of my degree, I embarked on what was considered at the time another niche area of study: children's literature. Unlike some, I didn't believe it required any less skill to write, or analyse, than adult fiction. The plots often had ancient foundations – myths, fairy tales, legends – as well as a focus on family relationships and identity issues, topics that underpin many stories for adults too. The course was stimulating, taking me back through childhood favourites and introducing me to new authors. Just a few weeks ago, I came across the short story and commentary that I wrote for my end-of-topic assessment at the bottom of a box in the loft. It's the tale of Sam Stevens, a 12-year-old overshadowed by an older sibling, who is cast as Little Red Riding Hood in a play put on by her local drama group. During the performance, she escapes into the fictional world of the play, where she feels important and valued. It's clear from the critical evaluation which I had to write alongside the story that I consciously based the real-life setting close to home, but reading it now, I'm astonished that I failed to notice how neatly the psychological elements of the story fitted into my own life. The nearest I came was when I explained in my evaluation:

Whilst I was aware, at the age of eight, that plays were not 'real' in a deterministic sense, they came alive in a different area of my consciousness. I always felt the sense of a liberated living force once the words left the page. I used to dream about plays metamorphosing and growing during a performance. I decided, therefore, to write from my own experiences, and to set the realistic side of the story in the drama group of my childhood.

Once Sam enters the 'forest', fiction takes over. By this point, she is no longer simply acting the role of Little Red Riding Hood. Instead, she becomes the red-robed rebel and heads off into the pine trees. Rereading the commentary, I'm reminded why I chose this landscape. Having just returned from my first and only skiing holiday, my mind was full of the sharp winds and shadowy forests of the Italian Alps. I've not thought about that trip for years. Probably because there are no cheerful mementos to remind me. No photos of me, just turned 21, grinning *en piste* in my ski gear. All I have is a letter from a friend in which he entreats me to spill the beans on any 'extremely awkward moments'. That jogs my memory. Ah yes, *that* holiday. No wonder I buried the story in a box in the loft.

It was a mortifying few weeks. I'd travelled to Italy with my ex-boyfriend and his family. They were all big skiers and he'd invited me to join them months earlier. All the arrangements had been made; the balance paid. Then, just before the trip, I told him I wanted to end our relationship. That I'd found someone else. As soon as we split up, my university friends shunned me. I was ignored, cast out overnight by people I'd lived and laughed with for nearly three years. Apart from a couple of dear friends who stuck by me, the rest hardly ever spoke to me again.

To his credit, my ex didn't withdraw the offer of the holiday. All this time later, I can't think why. Perhaps he thought we'd get back together. Perhaps I went to appease him – or my own sense of guilt. Was the siren song of snow and forests and mountain air just too strong? I don't remember. But it was a dark, painful time. I cried at night on the phone to my new boyfriend and hid my distress during the day. And I started to scribble down notes about a girl who escapes her friends and family, and her own sense of worthlessness, by walking out into the forest.

The notes grew into a short story and, as I wrote, the play inside the story came alive, digesting Sam, who felt surrounded by a 'palpitating, living body'. Trapped in the fairy-tale world, she realised she was following someone else's path rather than forging her own. The tale ended with Sam's return to the real world to take charge of her own life, even though she recognised a story for herself would be 'a challenging prospect'.

It was to be the last creative piece I wrote until I began the notes for this book. In the intervening 25 years I busied myself encouraging young people – first my students, then my own children – to develop their creativity. Immersed in their imaginative worlds, I forgot my protagonist's resolve to tell her own story in her own voice. And at no point did I ever stop to wonder what happened to the creative lass who dreamed about plays that came alive, who wrote poetry about dead, jerking dunnocks and the woman who fed the feral pigeons, or short stories where vergers buried stray dogs in windswept graveyards and a young girl lost and found herself in the forest.

My children's literature course culminated in Sam's story. The following year, during my secondary Postgraduate Certificate in Education (PGCE), I rolled up my sleeves and tackled children's literature hands-on, creating a scheme of work for 11- and 12-year-olds on Robert Westall's *The Wind Eye*. The story is based on the life of Saint Cuthbert, Bishop of Lindisfarne and hermit on the island of Inner Farne. Reading and creating activities on the book strengthened my relationship with the North East landscape and its history. My hope was that the saint's life on the Northumberland coast and the story of the founding of Durham Cathedral would engage the kids, drawing them deep into a sense of place the way the mosses and meres of *The Weirdstone of Brisingamen* had lured me in.

Westall was familiar with both Cheshire and Durham, his life's course having been sketched out in reverse to my own. Born in North Shields, Northumberland, in 1929, he studied fine art at Durham University. In 1960, he moved to live near Northwich in Cheshire, 3 miles from my childhood home. He started teaching at Sir John Deane's Grammar School and retired in 1985 (by which time it had become a sixth form college), six years before I walked through the doors. In 1993 he died of pneumonia, a few weeks before I sat my A levels. I wish I'd known he was there, just down the road in Magpie Antiques, the shop he opened when he retired from teaching. Perhaps writing or revising a chapter while he waited for the next customer. Now, reading his biography, *The Making of Me*, I warm to his frankness and verve. I think we'd have found a lot to talk about.

Like me, Westall was a late starter in publishing terms. His first book, *The Machine Gunners*, was published in 1975 – the year I was born. He wrote the manuscript on exercise books taken from the college stationery cupboard and it went on to win the Carnegie Medal. This first success unlocked a storm of creativity, and his second children's book, *The Wind Eye*, was published only a year later when he was 47, the age I am as I write this chapter. The time-slip story follows a Cambridge family: Bertrand, his two daughters and his wife, Madeleine, and her son, holidaying on the Northumberland coast. En route to their cottage they visit Durham Cathedral, where Madeleine steps on Saint Cuthbert's tomb in a moment of defiance, initiating a series of encounters with the long-dead saint that rock the whole family.

Saint Cuthbert has long been notorious for his alleged misogyny. However, early accounts suggest he had a good relationship with women. It was only centuries later that gynophobic stories about the saint proliferated, such as the legend of the line of Frosterley marble at the back of the cathedral nave, supposedly laid to prevent women approaching his shrine, and tales of tragic consequences for those women who disobeyed his edict. But cautionary tales don't stop Madeleine placing her shoe on the stone and declaring "'Women's Lib forever!'"

I have a certain amount of sympathy for her irreverence. By the time I encountered Cuthbert (or Cuddy, as I came to know him), I'd already crossed the Frosterley line into gendered space and sung in the choir stalls, but I stopped short of trespassing on his tomb.

A Saint's Life
I met him through music.
I called him to be my guide.
I blessed and glorified him.
I entreated him to heal my doubt
And resurrect my faith.

Bishop and hermit. My holy man. I followed you through tempest and battle, through plague and healing. To Lindisfarne, Island of Tides, Island of Prayer. To your ring of stone on Inner Farne. I watched you command the waves and die in your sanctuary. I fled from the fury of the Northmen with your incorrupt body.

I was there a thousand years ago when your bones were laid to rest in Durham. I stood beside your shrine. Joined the celebration of your life, heard your story raised up to the ribbed vaults.

Saint Cuthbert. Your words. Your music.
The most spiritual choral experience of my life.

December 1996: Durham University Choral Society perform the world premiere of Will Todd's oratorio, *Saint Cuthbert*. Composed for the millennium of the Diocese of Durham (founded in 995 when the saint's coffin was brought to the city), it has been sung in concert only once before, last year, with a smaller orchestral ensemble. Durham-born Todd's music, with lyrics by fellow north-easterner Ben Dunwell, is so deeply rooted in local history that singing it makes my entire body ring. It fills me with the same connective force I felt at the top of Loughrigg Fell. Music as conduit. Like *Resurre* – Cuthbert's funeral boat that sends Bertrand and his family deep into the saint's past in *The Wind Eye* – the oratorio sings me back in time.

Back to Inner Farne, to Cuddy's raw, eremitic life inside his wall of rough stones and turf. A monastic life with much to recommend it. Silence. Music. Contemplation. All those years living wild on the edge of the world. His affinity with the solitude of the sea. There are few places better suited to expansive thinking than an island, especially one off the dashing Northumberland coast. On the day my son became a teenager we stood together on the shingle in Suffolk looking out past the breakers and I asked him how the sea made him feel. "Small," he replied. I thought it a wise answer, though the sea also speaks to me of possibilities. In the face of the waves, salt-wind and limitless horizon, I am a braver and bolder version of myself.

The austerity of Cuddy's life on Inner Farne holds a certain attraction too. Though I was fortunate in my upbringing in some respects, there was more than a hint of the ascetic about it: a strict moral code, fear of indulgence of any kind – especially the sin of sugar – and a fair amount of isolation. I grew up believing pleasure was sanctified only for worthy causes like helping others, intellectual endeavours or aesthetic creation. Childhood honed my sense of self-denial and self-reliance, both necessary qualities for an anchorite. Who knows, perhaps I'd have considered it, had I not been missing one fairly fundamental component.

Unlike me, Cuddy and his followers had no issues with faith. After his death, legends about the saint's deeds were passed down and his reputation grew. Saint Cuthbert could control the elements. The sea calmed at his bidding. He commanded the birds and the beasts. Sally, the younger of Bertrand's two daughters in *The Wind Eye*, witnesses some of these incidents. One night she watches Cuthbert wade up to his arms in the sea singing praises to God, and, when he emerges, otters play around his feet. Many legends mention this rapport with animals, and the saint is often referred to as an early conservationist, based on the special laws he's said to have instigated to protect eider ducks on Inner Farne. This legend seems to have originated in a twelfth-century biography of the saint. It added several new animal miracles to the Cuthbert corpus and was the first document to associate him with the eider, so there's some doubt about the veracity of the claim. But the connection endures through the Northumbrian term for this endearing bird: the Cuddy duck.

By the time I met the saint, I was already familiar with the landscape around Durham. During the months when I learned the oratorio and then taught *The Wind Eye* to my first classes, I grew fond of Cuddy and Lindisfarne too. It was a privilege to share my enthusiasm with students. I wonder if any of them, now in their mid-30s, many no doubt with children of their own, remember the legends, photos and maps we studied; the Celtic bookmarks we drew; our time-travelling adventures with Bertrand, Madeleine and family on the Northumberland coast; the fact that Durham was founded when Cuthbert's body came to rest in our little crook of river over a thousand years ago. I guess I'll never find out what they took from the lessons, but I know I carried Cuddy's story and an enduring love of the North East landscape and its birds away with me when I left.

After completing my PGCE, I applied for teaching jobs in and around the city. By this time, I had a steady boyfriend and after four years in Durham it felt more like home than anywhere I'd ever lived. I started work as an English teacher in September 1997, in a large secondary school just outside the city. It was a demanding job, especially in those first few years, but I was lucky enough to have a supportive head of department from whom I learned a great deal. I felt like I'd found my place in the world, living and teaching in the North East. By the beginning of the new millennium, my boyfriend Col was partway through his PhD and I was the main wage-earner. I felt strong and independent. As well as working full-time, I kept busy directing school shows: rehearsing dialogue, setting dance numbers, teaching my foemen to bare their steel (though their weapons looked uncommonly like bananas) against the rollicking band of buccaneers in *The Pirates of Penzance*. But behind the scenes, I was struggling to control my anxiety and depression. And it was getting worse.

I managed to hold it in at work; it was easy to forget myself when there were so many young people needing my attention. Once home though, it was a different matter. The smallest thing and I'd dissolve in floods of tears, and once I started it was hard to stop; often I couldn't even have told you why I was crying. I felt so low, so pathetic, so unable to cope that I was often immobilised for hours by the hopelessness of it all. Something felt badly wrong.

However instinctive I might have been at understanding and supporting others, I was atrocious at reading my own signs. That's what happens when life teaches you to deny the validity of your own experience. If it hadn't been for Col, who became increasingly concerned about me, I'm not sure I'd ever have figured out what was going on. One weekend away in Edinburgh, I was too depressed to leave our room. I cried solidly for two days. We had to abandon our climb up Arthur's Seat, where, unbeknown to me, Col planned to propose. I'd not find out about the failed proposal until many years later. When we got back to Durham, he persuaded me to get some help.

We'd begun to notice a cyclical pattern to my worsening bouts of depression and wondered if the pill, which I'd been on for several years, might be responsible. The doctor's response was emphatic: "I think that extremely unlikely!" But I came off it anyway and though the anxiety remained, my depression improved. Hugely and rapidly. I was so lucky I had a partner to support me; otherwise I'd have crumbled in the face of the doctor's disbelief. It wasn't as if I needed anyone else to gaslight me – I was an expert at that myself. I quickly forgot how bad my mental health had been on the Edinburgh trip as my subconscious put into practice the lessons I'd learned as a child. When faced with illness you don't understand:

Ignore

Repress

Forget

But if you'd suggested to me back then that I was struggling with long-term fatigue, anxiety and depression, that I split myself in two so I could distance myself from illness once I recovered – well, no one who knew me ever would have done. I'd have told you straight out to sod off, then pulled away, sharpish. Those episodes did not belong to me; they were slippery. And though I'm trying to remember and accept the tough bits, I often need help: "Tell me about it again. Go through it one more time," I ask, over and over. "Did it really happen like that?"

When I managed to squeeze in the time and energy for other activities, Col and I would head out of the city. My birding journal reminds me we saw fulmars and kittiwakes one March off Filey Brigg in North Yorkshire and learned to identify razorbills, guillemots and gannets just down the coast at Bempton Cliffs; watched linnets, redpolls and goldfinches at Gibside in the Derwent Valley; exulted for days over the turquoise flare of bee-eaters in Bishop Middleham Quarry; heard wood warblers in Hamsterley Forest on a May afternoon when the air was coconut-soft with gorse.

Ah! Halcyon memories of our early birding trips… into which the incident with the cock pheasant slams with unwelcome force. All we saw was a russet streak as the witless pheasant tried to run straight across all six lanes of the A1 at once. To be fair, it was a surprisingly successful attempt. The pheasant made it all the way to the final lane before we hit it at 70 miles per hour.

A sharp crack. A rush of guilt and regret. Not that there was a lot we could have done, but we'd ended a life and we felt bad. At the next petrol station, Col got out to survey the damage. He gave me such a peculiar look that I jumped out to join him. There, poking out of the car radiator, were two scaly feet.

Good grief! Whatever next? We couldn't drive home with a pheasant sticking out of our Citroën ZX. So he took a firm grip on the legs and pulled. Up came a dead but seemingly undamaged cock pheasant in an effortless reveal like a rabbit out of a hat. The petrol forecourt was busy and by now our impromptu magic show had attracted quite a bit of attention. The audience seemed somewhat baffled by Col's coup de grâce and we were caught between embarrassment and hysterics. We stowed the hefty pheasant in the boot and drove home.

We should have left it at that. But it seemed such a shame to waste the delicious, plump-breasted pheasant, especially as we suspected its inability to follow the Green Cross Code would cost us hundreds of pounds we didn't have. So I rang Granny – the family roadkill oracle. She was undeterred by our tale and full of practical wisdom: "The first thing to do is to put a nick in the anus…"

After this opening gambit, I was treated to a forensic description of how to prep the unfortunate bird. But we were at the frayed end of a long day and we both knew the pheasant had beaten us. *We'll pluck the next one*, we thought as we dropped it head-first in the outside bin.

The most memorable entry in my early birding journal returns me to the Island of Tides. On this special Lindisfarne trip, we saw short-eared owls, brent geese, whooper swans, red-breasted mergansers and, of course, Cuddy ducks. We debated the identity of grebes in the sea ('red-necked or Slavonian?'), trudged through driving horizontal rain and sheltered in a succession of steamy hides with other soggy birders. Drying out by the fireside in Bamburgh after a deluge of a day on Holy Island, we ordered dinner, but I'd noticed Col struggling with his roast lamb, which was not at all normal. The reason for his lack of appetite soon became clear, when halfway through the main course he got down on one knee and held out the ring he'd kept in his pocket all day, waiting for the right time. He looked up at me and I answered the easiest question I'd ever been asked.

It was a magical moment and our waitress was delighted. She congratulated us loudly in front of the whole restaurant, then offered us free drinks. I was flummoxed to find myself the centre of attention. Col kept his cool and ordered a glass of port. I panicked. Hummed and hawed. Then, to my eternal embarrassment and our waitress's utter bemusement, I asked for a cup of tea.

By the summer of 2002, my new fiancé was nearing the end of his PhD and applying for jobs in government science. Almost all the departments were based in and around London. He began working for the Home Office in the November and moved into a rented room in St Albans, 215 miles south of our house in Durham. He and I were a unit, so I never considered staying behind. I'd have followed him anywhere, even if it meant saying goodbye to my happy places, my job, my northern roots. I taught on until the end of the Michaelmas term, packing up the house in the evenings, tearing myself away from our anarchic first garden, from the fields out back that brimmed with skylarks in spring and summer, from the River Browney where we'd linger at dusk watching Daubenton's bats swooping low under the bridges. By New Year I was ready (or so I told myself) – hardened off, bare-rooted – for the move Down South.

I find myself in an unfamiliar landscape: soft undulations, seeping mounds where I'd imagined mountains. My companion on this inaugural tour, my terse consultant, leads me up and down the modest inclines and shallow dips. I don't belong here, I try to say.

The native tongue is impenetrable, austere, frictionless – villous atrophy, malabsorptive, transglutaminase – the words slide in and, finding little purchase, slip back out again without trace. But I decode enough to see the terrain is disappointing, the dimensions unambitious; there are no peaks here worth scaling. Mine is a flattened landscape and its inadequate contours fold neatly into my life, a physical and emotional symbiosis as the landscape writes me, meekly, across the screen.

Flatlands

A cold coming we had of it that January, just the worst time of year to take a journey. The weather was sharp, the days short, the sun farthest off, in the very dead of winter. The temperature plummeted to −5 degrees Celsius. As we drove down the Great North Road from one rented house to another five hours south, it seemed nothing and everything had changed. The southern landscape looked as uninspiring to me as it had done to Arthur Young, Secretary of the Board of Agriculture, two centuries earlier when he wrote:

> To those, who consider picturesque beauty as an object of pursuit and pleasure, Hertfordshire will appear deficient in these grand scenes of Nature, in very extensive rivers and stupendous mountains.

Like Young, I was used to seeking the extensive and stupendous in places where nature appears raw and exposed. Hertfordshire flatly refused to meet my expectations. Where fenland meets chalkland there is neither level plain nor rolling heights but an uneasy combination of the two, a neither here nor there. Driving past copses and arable fields on the edge of our new town, I felt alienated by this self-contained land whose spirit seemed as deflated as its paltry contours. No wildness here. I'd left all that behind me in the North.

When we arrived at the new house, we discovered the heating had been off for weeks. The ancient boiler was broken and the pipes had frozen, so there wasn't any water. Knackered and cross, we gave up on the day and bedded down, wriggling deep into our sleeping bags, hats pulled tight over our ears. Hitchin had not endeared itself to us thus far. Next morning, we managed to find a plumber who fixed the boiler, and in the blink of 11 hours we had running water. Col returned to work the following day while I sat in a strange, cold house in a strange, cold town. Back in Durham my classes would be starting their first lesson of the week with their new teachers. I felt lonely and very far from home.

January was December in reverse. After weeks packing up our old life, now I unpacked and tried to get acquainted with a new one. By the first weekend I'd emptied most of the boxes, so we headed back up the A1 to the nearest RSPB reserve. Not far enough north for my liking, but at least we'd escaped the home counties and crossed over into Bedfordshire, which sounded a little less southern to my ear than Hertfordshire. The Lodge reserve at Sandy lies on the Greensand Ridge, a narrow sandstone escarpment that runs through Buckinghamshire, Bedfordshire and Cambridgeshire. It wasn't as wild as Druridge Bay (our last birding trip before we left the North East), but there were rumours of waxwings and a firecrest had been seen in the pines. Neither species appeared, but we enjoyed our day and the reserve became one of our favourite haunts. We saw a couple of lifers there that first year – crossbills in March and breeding spotted flycatchers at the beginning of May.

Life was busy in those first few months. I started applying for sixth form jobs and we planned our wedding. At night I'd often travel up north: a roving, longing dreamer. Mornings found me befuddled, a little bereft, wrenching my attention back to making a life for us in the South. I rarely dream myself back to Durham these days. My last visit in person was nearly two decades ago. Perhaps my aching northern core, disregarded for so long, has quietly withered away. I want to know if anything remains from those days, so I close my eyes and reach inside, dig deep. I'm kissed by pinkness and light.

Pinkness: Washing up at the kitchen sink in Crossgate Moor on the outskirts of Durham, distracted by the saccharine pink of the tree mallow at the end of the overgrown lawn, a shade I so disliked elsewhere, yet these lavish blooms redeemed it. It was the only flower in the grassy wilderness when we arrived. For years after I left, pink tree mallows whispered me back to that garden.

Light: An ordinary day walking across the college car park when a sunbeam winked on the path in front of me. Just that. A tiny spot lit by a shaft that pierced the tree canopy, but the brightness struck me with Cupid's arrow. I was illuminated from within like a page of the Lindisfarne Gospels. Beauty. Knowledge. A final epiphany. The last time I experienced unadulterated childlike wonder.

Pinkness. Light. A tingle in my nose. A prickle of tears. Though I hardly ever feel the pull northwards anymore, part of me still remembers.

At the end of February, I was offered a job at a sixth form college in Cambridge. Life settled into a fast-paced rhythm. The hour-long commute, my daily ascent of Hills Road (a derisory appellation for what passed for a hill in one of the flattest counties in the UK), my days teaching English literature, language and media studies. At weekends and on holidays we travelled further afield, getting to know Minsmere and Dunwich Heath in Suffolk (our first Dartford warblers and nightjars), Titchwell Marsh (fond memories of Sammy the black-winged stilt, first sighted back in Druridge Bay in 1993) and Holme Bird Observatory on the Norfolk coast where we saw yellow-browed and barred warblers. We explored Fen Drayton, Fowlmere, Paxton Pits and Wicken Fen in Cambridgeshire and saw our first smew – with its 19 companions – in the Lee Valley.

Looking back, it surprises me how often we drove out of our adopted county in those early years. Quite why I never considered exploring on foot, I'm not sure. Even when we married and moved to the edge of town, just a few minutes' walk from a small Wildlife Trust wetland reserve, I don't think I registered the existence of nature in the local area. Hitchin was a suburban place to sleep and eat and dance and sing. It seemed a rootless landscape, not somewhere to go looking for the wild.

Perhaps unsurprisingly, my records from this period list only the most important information – the birds. The rest of life is a matter of conjecture until we discover Col's old diaries on a geriatric computer we retired to the cupboard years ago. His daily entries remind me we travelled the world sampling Hitchin's cuisine (our favourite local restaurants were Australian, Thai, Greek and Mexican), sharing a main meal where we could get away with it, drinking tap water so we could afford to eat out. We joined the local choir and am-dram group, and started ballroom and Latin lessons in the hope we'd not embarrass ourselves when we took to the floor for our wedding dance. As our social circle expanded, we'd pop down the pub after choir and spend our weekends with friends: sharing meals, playing board games and chatting in a replay of our student days in Durham. When I survey the smoking ruins of my social life now – post-kids, post-Covid, so much more affected by debilitating anxiety these days – I'm surprised at how much time I chose to spend in the company of other people back then.

Col and I were married in St Mary's Church in Hitchin at the end of the summer term. Ours was an idiosyncratic wedding. There was more laughter, someone said, than they'd ever heard at a wedding before. Mid-service, Jane the vicar spirited us all away to the woods in her sermon on love and the tawny owl. She asked us to consider the owl's call – *Tu-whit Tu-who* – though in reality you might hear it rather as *kee-wik* (the female's call) and *hu-hoo* (the male's answer). Jane's point was that one owl was not enough. It took two to perform this love song.

If we ignore the fact that Shakespeare's strigine impersonation originates from *Love's Labour's Lost*, possibly not the ideal play to cite at a wedding, and that the tawny owl has historically been considered a symbol of bad luck and death, then it was a thoughtful and perfectly apt analogy. An interweaving of our shared love of music and birds. While we signed the register, a small choir of family and friends sang Fauré's *Cantique de Jean Racine*, then we left the church with a hop and a skip to the riotous strains of Lefébure-Wély's *Sortie in Eb Major*. Later that evening our practice finally paid off as we rumbaed to the bittersweet saxophone from *Miss Saigon*. All eyes were on us, the music was achingly beautiful, and we danced like it was the last night of the world.

So, there you go. I'm 29. Happily married. Teaching full-time at a renowned sixth form college. Busy social life. Let's leave it at that, shall we? I'd rather we ignored the other threads running through the diaries. But the writing task I've set myself – to own my life honestly and effect a reconciliation between the both of me – won't let me sidestep the persistent references to insomnia; the fight to get up for work in the morning when sleeping pills turned my mind to treacle; the gripping, sickening anxiety; the way the busyness of life often sapped more strength than I had, leaving me shattered, lacking even the energy to get out of bed, let alone sit in the garden or walk in the countryside.

This kind of fatigue is a strange mistress, especially when you deny its potency. The world recedes. Rising from the sofa preoccupies you for what seems like hours and in that performance there's always a shadow of self-indulgent histrionics. Everyone else manages, everyone else can get up at will, so why the fuck can't you? Stairs become a formidable ascent to be scaled on hands and knees, preferably with assistance. That the body functions, that it manifestly *can* move, *can* climb, is self-evident, so why won't it? I avoided long-distance travel and unnecessary journeys. Even my daily commute could reduce me to a non-being, an absence, a sofa-pinioned, mind-fogged captive.

I fought this exhaustion on both physical and mental fronts. Severe fatigue wasn't supposed to be part of my life. My body didn't get ill like this. Sure, I got colds, the occasional bout of flu. I was prone to throat infections after years of using my voice all day long. But not the lingering, unpredictable, inexplicable stuff. That kind of illness was not and never could be me. Childhood had made me acutely sensitive to my own and other people's prejudices. The questions about why I got so tired, why I needed so many naps, the letter from a friend that asked 'What on earth is wrong with you? You are always getting strangely ill...'. Perhaps I'd become too familiar with seeing myself through other people's eyes, my long-term fatigue a puzzling character trait, an external sign of some secret personal weakness.

When my body succumbed, I'd detach, numbly retreating to wait it out, hiding those days, weeks, the occasional month when I felt less than. And when I eventually emerged, my dissociative memory came in handy. Within a matter of days, I could gloss over the empty periods with a respectable veneer of energy and forget my bed-bound alter ego. What exhaustion? What isolation? Perhaps someone had spent those days in that bed, but it sure as hell wasn't me. I locked those times up in a box with my childhood fears, beneath which lay the other lady in the other bed: the one I still want to run away from because being with her hurts me.

By the time I reached my early 30s, the decision about whether to have children preoccupied me. I knew Col wanted a family. His longing for kids lay, unspoken, between us. But I didn't. The thought of motherhood irritated me. Like an annoying itch between the shoulder blades that eluded any attempt at a gratifying scratch. I cared deeply for my students and enjoyed their company, most of the time. But kids of my own? I was destined to be a teacher, not a mother. I understood intellectual relationships with teenagers. But physical ones? With babies? And toddlers? Pregnancy, birth, breastfeeding? Nappies, crying, cuddling? It all sounded far too much like my biology lessons at school: those diagrams that laid out the female body in all its swelling fecundity, that chart listing all the unpleasant conditions and diseases caused by pregnancy and birth, scientific evidence of the myriad ways our bodies could malfunction and mobilise against us. I knew a little of the intractable female body first-hand and wished to know no more. I'd rather hoped I'd left such disagreeable topics behind me at A level when I dropped biology in favour of English.

For years I'd followed the premise that if motherhood was right for me, at some point I'd know. Now I wasn't so sure. I felt myself teetering at the top of a dangerous slope. Dally too close to the edge and... what if I fell over and lost my sense of self forever? What if I became permanently ill, unhappy, unreachable? The last thing I wanted was to have children and resent the decision. For it to change me. To lay all that on young shoulders. Like all other important decisions I'd made in life, I wanted to go in open-eyed and with an open heart. So it seemed I had little option but to wait...

And, eventually, my patience paid off. I'm not sure quite how and when I changed, when fear softened to gentle curiosity, a quiet dream, an unspoken desire, a shared plan. Those first couple of months of trying, all nerves and excitement; a few months more, a hopeful rhythm; the months running on, that stronger sense of our dual longing; my body-ache as we approached a year and I considered the irony that the decision

I'd waited so long to make may have been as unnecessary as our years of contraception. I looked into the possibility of a future without the need to fear what motherhood would make of me, a future that only a few years earlier would have brought me relief, and saw only heartache.

As our year of trying drew to a close we went to the doctor for advice. I know now that adenomyosis and untreated coeliac disease could have affected my fertility, but at the time I was undiagnosed and the tests came back clear. All attention turned to Col, whose little guys were absurdly plentiful but couldn't always be bothered to complete the job in hand. We laughed when the doctor told us. By then the results didn't seem to matter, because a holiday on an organic cattle farm in Suffolk had done the trick. Five happy May days by the sea, 80 bird species and long uplifting evenings with pillows tilting my hips, legs skywards against the wall (who knows if it worked but it amused us) and I was finally pregnant.

Like my mother before me, my health improved during pregnancy. I felt energetic and, by the end of the summer, decided I was well enough to audition for our next musical, *Calamity Jane*, even though I'd be well into the second trimester by production week. Neither Col nor I looked much like we had last time we'd performed the show a decade earlier in Durham. Instead of captivating the ladies as Lieutenant Danny Gilmartin, Col played Francis Fryer, the hapless male entertainer railroaded into performing in drag to placate the irate audience in Deadwood. While he flounced round the Golden Garter saloon in ginger wig, red evening dress and high heels, I donned fishnets and feathers as one of Adelaide Adams's nubile dancing girls, my bonny bump concealed behind a giant scarlet heart to avoid shattering the illusion.

Calamity Jane was the last time we performed in a theatre together. My few memories of the show are precious, not just because I danced every evening with Bumpy along for the ride, but because of the music. 'The Black Hills of Dakota' had been one of our favourite songs when we performed the show in Durham. The lyrics took me back to an American wilderness of pine forests and mountains; the call of home reminded me of my old life back up north. We sang it in harmony every night before bed, Col's cheek against my swollen belly, sharing our love of music and landscape with the new life growing inside me.

In later years, Black Hills became our family lullaby. One distressing day in A & E when our firstborn was still young and needed a blood test for a worrying rash, the nurse asked us if we knew anything that might calm our frightened baby. We started up the old harmony. The effect was immediate. Limbs relaxed, fear loosened its hold, the crying stopped. The nurse was astonished at the power of a simple song, but we knew this magic ran deep. Music was part of what bound us together as a family.

Col tried to give blood while we were at university. He fainted before he got as far as the chair. Many years later he accompanied me to a blood test and passed out again. The nurse looked at me. "Never have children with this man," she said.

I ignored her of course, but her advice comes back to me when we're planning for the birth. By 37 weeks, it's all gone a bit pear-shaped. Bumpy won't turn and scans reveal the reason: the cord is wrapped multiple times around its neck lashing it in place, head up like an unlucky coin toss. I'm booked in for a caesarean at 39 weeks. February turns snowy and deep drifts block the roads. Our lovely neighbours Lynne and Ruth offer to cart me to hospital in our shared wheelbarrow if I go into labour early.

I'm terrified by the prospect of a caesarean. I've never needed an operation before, so haven't had to face up to my phobia of doctors and hospitals. When the consultant tells me a vaginal birth is no longer an option, I go into shock. Antenatal appointments turn into distressing ordeals. I'm asked impossible questions:

"What's your name?"
"Address?"
"Date of birth?"

I'm sure I knew the answers once, but that bit of my brain is missing and my voice has shrunk to a whisper. The consultants are tall, impersonal, completely in control. I'm small – smaller – smallest like I'm shrinking too. The noises and lights in the hospital bewilder me. I come out of every appointment in floods of tears. The day of my caesarean gets ever closer.

I enter the operating theatre because I know there will be music. I've chosen it to save me. Col is with me, but he's a medical liability of his own, bless him. Within five minutes he is sat on the floor in the corner, feeling faint, surrounded by my midwives. When I sit there on the table; when they inject me with the epidural and top it up twice because I can still feel my legs; when they lie me down, block off my view with a sheet, cut and peer; I know I have made my choice. Allegri's *Miserere* is my agency.

I feel the pulling and know there is no escape. I couldn't avoid this moment, because I needed to save Bumpy, who is my responsibility. Music helps me hold on to this when I shake like a frightened kid when the panic sets in when I want to run run run away cry and fight scream and hide the music is there to lift me up and bring me down into my body again and the other body they're taking out of me that I can see purple and angry above the sheet.

I soar with the treble and, through the music, I see my son.

As a new mother I fought to be active but it was hard to deny that positivity and energy came at a significant price. Like all women in my maternal line, I struggled to breastfeed and within a few days developed postnatal depression. Col needed increasingly frequent periods off work to run the house and look after us. The doctor prescribed antidepressants but a deep-seated distrust of medicine cauterised my free will and the pills sat on the shelf at the top of the cupboard, unopened. History was repeating itself. Motherhood exacting its pound of flesh. I felt I was falling down a well – watching my good health in pregnancy, my ability to look after myself and my son receding, until they were mere pinpricks against the sky.

Despite misgivings in the past, I was now desperate to breastfeed. I'd not managed the home birth we'd planned.

Breastfeeding seemed the best way to recapture some of that fabled natural mother-and-baby bonding time. I knew it might be hard, especially after a caesarean. But evidence suggested it would be better for my son, so I persevered, even though my body couldn't wring out the milk and the poor bairn was hungry all the time. When I look back at photos, I can't help but cry. How did I not see how thin he was? Why didn't the health visitors tell me to jack it all in and give him a bottle? I feel I failed him by carrying on when I should have given up. But I thought it was my fault: that if I tried harder, it would get easier.

When he still hadn't regained his birth weight by five weeks, a senior health visitor came round and suggested we give him a bottle after every breastfeed. He downed the first within seconds and let out an almighty scream that subsided only when we gave him another. He gained 21 ounces that week – around three times the average weekly weight gain. Even then, I refused to give up. I expressed five times a day and used a supplementary feeding system to try and stimulate my flow. It never occurred to me as I taped the feeding tube to my breast and tucked the end beside my nipple in his eager mouth that my body was incapable of producing enough milk. That I could have given it every ounce of determination I possessed and he'd still have gone hungry.

I was persuaded to stop after three months when it became obvious to those around me that trying to breastfeed was damaging my mental health. My milk dried up almost immediately. Col took over the night feeds so I could sleep. Depression hit with a vengeance. I felt so guilty, as if, somehow, I hadn't been pulling my weight. The other mums I knew were still up feeding in the night, whereas I couldn't provide the milk or cope with the lack of sleep. It was another three months before

I started to feel a bit more normal. By then our days were filled with toddler music classes and outside play sessions. Life settled into a routine again.

The months passed. When I had spare time, I'd roam around Hitchin on Google Earth looking for land. I'd had this recurring dream for a while where I'd suddenly notice a gate at the end of our tiny garden leading to a hidden allotment just around the corner. With a greenhouse. And real vegetable beds. The garden of my dreams. Then, when our son Jamie was nearly 18 months old, a house in need of repair came on the market. It was in an area I'd always liked for its mature trees and quiet atmosphere, and the garden was one of the biggest on the estate at 9 metres by 13 metres. It was love at first sight. Not quite the wild third-of-an-acre I'd enjoyed as a child, but a step up from our current shady plot, the first garden we'd ever owned, where I learned painful lessons from figs and lupins about the importance of right plant, right place. By late summer we'd moved house. It was exciting to have an open sunny garden. I could see so much potential to create a family space where we could all play and grow together.

In September, I enrolled on a garden design course at a local adult education centre. There was no grand plan; it was simply my attempt to have a bit of me time. I wanted to see if I could reassemble the residue of what had once passed as a brain. It was great to be out of the house talking about plants and I felt in pretty good shape that autumn. Then in December we all came down with gastroenteritis. The boys recovered quickly, but I couldn't seem to shake it off. I waited, prevaricated for weeks (a particular talent of mine), but to no avail. Three months on, the unpleasant after-effects showed no signs of abating.

Reluctantly, I agreed it was sensible to get checked out, so I made an appointment to see the doctor.

I don't know what I was expecting from the results of the tests they recommended. A clear bill of health and the gastric symptoms to disappear soon afterwards perhaps. Certainly, I didn't expect to be diagnosed with coeliac disease. I was tested because my dad had been diagnosed five years earlier, but never dreamed I'd have inherited the condition from him. When the doctor phoned to tell me my blood test was positive and I'd need a biopsy for confirmation, I listened in disbelief. I was the family member without dietary requirements and immune complications. My personality was founded on being distinct from the physical restrictions, mental suffering and social isolation my mum's illness caused. I couldn't accept that it was my body we were talking about. Surely there'd been a mistake?

My first appointment with the gastroenterology consultant brought on all the usual feelings of animosity and fear. By this point, with perfect ironic timing, my stomach symptoms had gone. There seemed little reason for a gluten-free diet now I was better. I don't think anyone had told me that exhaustion was one of the main diagnostic features of the disease, or, if they had, I'd dismissed it because it clearly didn't apply to me. At one point in my medical records, the consultant writes 'on direct questioning however, she does admit to longstanding fatigue', which sounds about right. I imagine the only way he'd have got it out of me was under cross-examination.

By the second appointment I had my biopsy results – incontrovertible evidence of the extensive damage to my small intestine. The consultant explained how in patients with coeliac disease, the ingestion of gluten causes an immune reaction that attacks the villi, or finger-like projections, in the small intestine, flattening them and reducing their capacity to take up nutrients. Malabsorption can lead to vitamin and mineral deficiency and malnutrition. I'm not sure how much of it I took in. It was all too overwhelming. I felt angry and somehow diminished by association with the internal flatland he'd described. But in light of the damage revealed by the biopsy, I begrudgingly agreed to try a gluten-free diet for 12 months, still convinced I was asymptomatic. Once the year was up and I was much the same as ever, I reckoned I'd have pacified the wretched man and life could return to normal.

Three months into the new regime and I felt amazing. Changes were taking place in my 'asymptomatic' body. My energy levels were higher than I'd ever remembered. I was able to walk round a shopping centre without feeling like I was wading through the floor. I could make it to the end of a Latin dance class without the world swimming in and out of focus as I fought to stay upright. Best of all, I could engage more actively with my young son, playing on the floor and taking him into the garden rather than simply spectating from the sofa. Looking back over the previous 15 years, little details began to surface. The struggle to cope with the energy required for teaching (didn't everyone find it a tiring job?), my frequent inability to climb the stairs without assistance or rise before midday at the weekends, those intermittent days and weeks in bed (presumably other people just tried harder than I did to get on with life). I realised I hadn't been asymptomatic, just unaware of the harmful effects of the damage to my gut. It turned out I wasn't weak or pathetic. The results of my biopsy gave me a medical explanation for my exhaustion. I felt this was the beginning of a new life. Armed with a gluten-free diet, I approached my late 30s with more energy than I'd ever had and felt I'd conquered long-term fatigue for good.

Until 2006 there was a brutalist café complex at the summit of Mount Snowdon, supposedly described by the Prince of Wales as a 'carbuncle'. I'd have to agree, though on more than purely aesthetic grounds. Though many of my childhood holidays were spent walking and foraging in the Welsh hills above my grandparents' terraced house in Conwy or messing about on their boat in the estuary, we rarely followed the tourist trails. So I didn't have the pleasure of visiting Snowdon's café until I was in my early 20s. We'd walked up (me, Col and my cousins, aunt, dad and grandpa) and met Mum and Granny (the train travellers) at the top. Mum's stringent diet, which she followed to help with her ME/CFS symptoms, meant there was nothing in the café she could eat. Instead, she brought a Tupperware box filled with tinned fish, rice cakes, salad and, no doubt, a substantial slab of frillet, otherwise known as cooked millet fried with egg. We were luckier. Even though I sympathised, I still viewed her culinary concoctions with a mixture of pity and horror. I imagine I was looking forward to a hot meal – most likely I'd have chosen a cup of tea and all-day breakfast on what turned out to be a particularly chilly Easter afternoon.

The café had the usual welcoming signs on the tables: 'Only food and drink purchased here can be consumed on these premises' or some such edict. Generally, a polite request was all it took for venues to make an exception under the circumstances, providing

Mum agreed to keep her Tupperware tucked discreetly beneath the table. And on this occasion there were eight other people in our party buying lunch. But the waitress who served us – in classic carbuncle style – had the empathy of a boil. She refused outright to let Mum join us at the table. Further explanation provoked only further rudeness, so Mum had little choice but to take her cold lunch outside and sit on a bench in the summit wind. Inside the warm café, we finished our meal. Then we got the hell out of there.

We've moved on a decade or so now from that lunch in Snowdon's carbuncle. Old drama, new parts. I surreptitiously check my script, only to find I've been cast as the difficult customer, a role for which I'm sure I didn't audition. The part is not at all to my liking. It appears I'm expected to question the serving staff, speak to the chef and, on occasions, send food back pending further enquiries. But whereas Mum seemed to inflate with indignation when people were rude to her, having to fight my corner with strangers makes me want to dissolve. I'd rather eat my own words and vanish in a mouthful of silence than have to ask exactly where and how my food was prepared and cooked. Unfortunately, once I've taken centre stage as the coeliac at the table, I don't have much choice. I could, of course, avoid the scene altogether. I could shirk family celebrations, decline meals with friends and make my excuses at special events. And I do. Often.

Or I could join the Tupperware crew. The covert extract-a-sandwich-under-the-table-and-hope-no-one's-looking brigade. Or accept that I need to badger the catering staff or my host, then trust they know what they're doing. Like the time I was assured my meal would be gluten-free by the chef when I phoned before a conference at a four-star hotel, and again by the waitress at the table. They were almost right. But the spicy wheat-based coating on the chips was enough to make me ill for weeks. I must also hope no one blames me for asking questions intended to prevent my immune system from attacking itself. Sometimes people do.

"I hope you didn't mind me asking you about cross-contamination," I enquired gingerly when a colleague who'd cooked a meal for me seemed a tad pissed off. They looked me in the eye and my heart sank. I knew what was coming. "Actually, I did. Yes."

Oh. Well. That's me told then. I imagine they thought me an ungrateful, paranoid hypochondriac. But I know how difficult it can be to avoid even the tiniest speck of gluten from my own attempts to cater for my dad in the five years before I was diagnosed. And coeliac disease is a lifelong autoimmune condition, not an allergy or food intolerance or a faddy diet. For someone with the condition, that tiny speck need only be the size of a crumb, or smaller, and we're in trouble. It could be stuck in the butter or lurking at the bottom of the toaster, which is why coeliacs are advised not to share condiments and to have their own food preparation spaces, toasters and chopping boards.

If I make a mistake, my immune system reacts by mounting a wholesale attack on my body. Within an hour or two I know I've been glutened. My belly bloats and a tight band of pain constricts my upper abdomen. It lasts for several days and is not relieved by painkillers. Eyesight is next. Focusing becomes tricky; the world seems alternately too vivid, then dingy and distant. It doesn't take long before my limbs increase in weight, brain fog descends and I feel like I've come down with flu. By this point, functioning is practically impossible.

Last time I was fed gluten without my knowledge, I ended up in bed for a fortnight. Then, on the way back from taking my son to school on my first day out of the house, I almost passed out. Fortunately, I was walking beside a parent with a baby in a pushchair. Clinging to the handle with my head lowered, I realised I hadn't recovered as much as I'd thought. And, without a biopsy, it's impossible to know how much damage an exposure has had on our under-researched, internal landscapes. Coeliac UK cautions that 'even tiny amounts of gluten may cause people with coeliac disease to have symptoms in the short term, and gut damage long term'. Potential long-term gut damage with all the repercussions that might involve – not just, as some people think, a couple of days feeling a bit dodgy. Eating out in restaurants and other people's houses is a game of Russian roulette and, though I might get lucky, I don't find it a particularly enjoyable experience.

So, if you bake for me, I'll smile and appreciate your thoughtfulness. But unless you cook in a gluten-free kitchen, I won't eat your cakes. And if you receive my polite "No thank you" with understanding, I'll never forget your kindness.

Grounded

More than a decade after my diagnosis, I write a list of the food and drink I miss most as a coeliac. It begins with beer.

> Guinness: Mum drank stout when trying to breastfeed me. I didn't get much milk but I've always loved dark beer.
> Desperados: To accompany hot chillies, sombreros and turkey fajita Christmas dinners with friends.
> Doom Bar: My sunset beer of choice at the end of a day's walk.

Guinness. Desperados. Doom Bar. These old pals are much missed. Though the range of gluten-free beer has widened considerably in the last few years, I still pine for these once familiar friends. Then there's sausage rolls, egg custards, profiteroles, iced buns, doughnuts, Danish pastries, cookie dough ice cream, cheddar cheese and Branston Pickle sandwiches on proper soft granary bread. Oh my! The stuff of salivating daydreams, so different from my real dreams...

which always begin after the eating...
missing out on the taste...
just as it's sinking in...
what I've done...

then two fingers down my throat and I dream I'm throwing up in a bathroom somewhere, purging my sins. Sometimes I'm in the downstairs toilet of my childhood bungalow in Cheshire. This is the moment I wake in a cold sweat. It takes a few minutes to digest the fact I've left my glutenous transgressions and their consequences behind in my sleep.

I can drink gluten-free beer and make my own sausage rolls of course, but it's not quite the same. And then there's bread: staple food for millennia. Now that deserves a substantial chapter all of its own. Gluten-free loaves might be better than they were a decade ago when you needed air-tight packaging to keep the slices from crumbling to dust before they reached your plate, but the cardboard taste and texture are still a far cry from the soft gluten bread I remember, a fact corroborated by family members who eat both. *No problem*, I thought in the early days, *I'll just bake my own.* As a child, I lived down the road from a Roberts Bakery. The warm yeasty smell that enveloped us as we stopped at the traffic lights beside the bread factory signalled the most wholesome homecoming in the world. Once I left home, I often made brown loaves based on my granny's recipes, and sourdough with a yeast starter that had been passed between friends for years. I knew I'd need to get used to new flours and new techniques, but really, how hard could it be?

Ha! You know the three little pigs? Well, those first two dimwits would have lived to see another day if they'd built with my focaccia instead of straw and sticks. No matter how hard the big bad wolf had huffed and puffed, their gluten-free houses would have remained standing. I could have started a cottage industry for porcine builders. But no little pigs came calling, so I made only the one brick. I didn't need to hear the clang as it bounced off the bottom of the brown bin to know I'd not delivered the soft crumb the recipe had promised. And my subsequent efforts weren't much better. I had no choice but to accept the new reality: my days of breaking bread with friends were over. My bread was unbreakable.

Since diagnosis, I've become adept at pastry (shortcrust and rough-puff); I can bake a light Victoria sponge and knock up a tasty batch of cheese straws. For Col's thirty-seventh birthday I made a gluten-free gingerbread house complete with stained-glass windows and internal lighting. When the kids were younger, I constructed a chocolate treasure chest, Shaun the Sheep, rainbow cakes and a piano, all from gluten-free vanilla or chocolate sponge. But I still can't bake a tolerable loaf. If anyone tells you their homemade gluten-free bread is soft, light and delicious, they're lying. Or they're a far better cook than me. If so, please give them my congratulations and send them my way. It's been over a decade since I've had a decent slice of bread.

Adopting a gluten-free diet, which is the only treatment for coeliac disease, has many health benefits. It's likely to have reduced my chances of developing osteoporosis and, after 11 years on the diet, my risk of developing lymphoma and small bowel cancer should be no greater now than that of the general population. As well as the diet significantly improving my energy levels, when we tried for a second child not long after I was diagnosed, I conceived within the first few days. The fact I gave birth naturally was nothing to do with the diet, but I breastfed my daughter for

11 months without any issues. I breastfed her. Me. As she'd often say once she learned to talk: "I do it by self." I'm proud of that. Our physical bond felt so intimate, so precious. Her milky kisses woke a tender part of me that had been sleeping for longer than I could remember.

But there are lasting challenges too. When I went for a second biopsy, two years after my diagnosis, the results showed persistent partial villous atrophy, or wasting of the villi. A slight improvement on the initial results, my consultant said, but not the significant internal recovery he'd expected. He intimated it was because I was 'non-compliant' with the diet. I could feel my hackles rising.

"How on earth can I be non-compliant?" I wanted to yell at him across the desk. "What more must I do to recover?"

I lived in a gluten-free house, never ate out and had almost completely forsaken what social life I had left as a new mum. None of my friends invited me to join the newly organised, socially active cake club. Can't say I blame them. It would have been like inviting a celibate teetotaller to a raunchy house party. But I missed out on conversation and social bonding. My confidence waned. I slipped further and further outside my friendship circle.

I'd always assumed, as is my wont, that the extent to which my diagnosis affected my lifestyle, confidence and mental health was down to my own personal brand of hyperreaction, especially as hardly anyone else seemed to think it was a big issue after the first few weeks. "You'll be fine," one of my friends reassured me with the kindest of intentions when she heard about my diagnosis. "You're interested in good food and cooking from scratch." Initially, that's what I thought too. I reckoned once I'd adjusted to managing without, given my eating habits were a frugal hangover from my childhood anyway, I'd not be missing much. I completely underestimated the role of food in human bonding and relationships.

As I researched for this book, I found many studies that set my experiences in context, such as the 2013 paper 'Living with coeliac disease: a grounded theory study', which notes that the condition 'has been linked with elevated levels of psychological distress, including depression, anxiety and social phobia'. Researchers cited 'loss of the former diet, changed personal and social identities, loss of social confidence and loss of social activities' as the main causes of 'grief' for coeliacs.

I'm certainly a different person since my diagnosis. I don't like venturing out into social situations. At home I'm just me. Out there in the world where food is involved – and it so often is – I'm a coeliac, constantly having to turn down, check or risk what I once took for granted. Earlier in the week, Col came in from work and told me that he and a colleague had wandered through London and found a little Malaysian café where they'd stopped for lunch. I can't remember what that feels like. To walk through a town or city and know you can pop in anywhere to eat. Not to carry your own food with you all the time or pass bakery windows flaunting doughnuts, bread and butter pudding, Cornish pasties, chicken pies... knowing there's not a single item in the shop you can eat. Sometimes it feels like living in an alternate reality. Sometimes I just stay at home.

Social integration is centred around rituals of eating. From the earliest days when hearth and home meant fire, family, friends and food, we've developed ways of celebrating and strengthening relationships that focus on feasting. Wedding breakfasts, harvest suppers, christening buffets, barbeques, Easter lunches, picnics, work meals, Christmas dinners. I find these occasions an unwelcome reminder that I exist outside social circles in a subtle but fundamental way. If I decide to attend, every event requires meticulous planning in advance, often with multiple emails to catering companies to arrange special food or get permission to bring my own.

Then there's smaller social gatherings. We'd intended to carry on going round for meals at friends' houses, but soon realised it was less painful to decline invitations than to accept. Just after my diagnosis, we were invited round for dinner with old friends. They were lovely and worked so hard to accommodate me, taking note of cross-contamination advice and checking ingredients in advance. We were just about to start the main course when they realised the butter in my dinner had come from the same pack they'd used to butter their bread. Such an easy mistake to make. I was grateful they'd realised and told me but, of course, I couldn't eat the meal. I was mortified. I cried, then felt worse for making a fuss. In the decade that has passed since then, I don't think I've accepted another dinner invitation.

It's important to me that Col and the kids aren't restricted too much, so when we're invited out to eat, I usually stay behind or head off for a walk. I remember one afternoon when I stalked the beach in Kessingland in a howling storm, wallowing in pathetic fallacy. The alternative was to join our big group of friends – four families in all – in the fish and chip restaurant, smelling the scampi, cod and chips, watching everyone else eat, sucking on my own self-pity. *Much better*, I thought, *to walk off my foul mood in the battering rain and avoid spoiling their fun.*

And it's not just social gatherings. Coeliac disease restricts me in other ways too. I've left the UK only twice since I was diagnosed. On the first occasion a friend won ferry tickets to France and offered them to us. It seemed churlish not to accept. We had a lovely week camping in the Vendée. Jamie was two and a half. He enjoyed the pool and waterslides at the campsite. We whiled away the afternoons at the beach and wandered the boulevards of nearby Saint-Jean-de-Monts. Patisseries were out of bounds for me, of course. No baguettes, eclairs, pains au chocolat or croissants.

We'd printed off a sheet of information about coeliac disease in French to take into restaurants, but most of the waiters raised eyebrows or shrugged once they'd read it. International sign language for "Dunno what you're talking about mate." The cafés and bistros along the seafront served pastries and brioches. They specialised in seafood, including my favourite: moules marinières. Potentially gluten-free, but off the menu without assurances about cross-contamination. We built sandcastles downwind of bouillabaisse, platters of *fruits de mer*, *le préfou* (a local garlic bread) and a French soup of other tantalising aromas. Later, we stocked up on gluten-free supplies at the *supermarché*. The pasta we bought melted, then resolidified into a dense, viscous mass at the bottom of the saucepan. Already struggling to cope with the volatile inner workings of early pregnancy, I forced down chunks of yellow flab doused in *sauce tomate*. My stomach rebelled and my nose returned wistfully to the beachfront.

It was worse on the ferry journey home. We'd travelled out overnight, so there was no need to eat. On the return trip, a grim combination of morning sickness, seasickness and a day with hardly any food, as the only gluten-free fare they could muster was one small pot of yoghurt despite my enquires in advance, led to the worst nausea I've ever experienced. I recovered soon enough, but it became clear that travelling as a coeliac was an extremely efficient way to lose weight. This was confirmed a few years later when we were invited on a two-day cruise with extended family. The company's grandiose gluten-free assurances failed at the first hurdle. I was cautiously optimistic on the first morning. Five full breakfasts arrived for the six of us, but when I enquired about my gluten-free breakfast, the waiting staff seemed uncertain. Eventually, they brought out a plate of beans, bacon, egg and black pudding. Having been assured once that the breakfast was gluten-free, I now faced a dilemma. Should I eat it, on the assumption that this was the first gluten-free black pudding I'd ever come across? Or make a nuisance of myself by questioning staff again, following my gut instinct? Despite my loathing of attracting attention, I asked them to check again. They took the plate away with rather bad grace, leaving me feeling like a demanding diva. After a few minutes the plate returned. Minus the black pudding. It wasn't gluten-free, they'd decided. By this point, I'd reached the end of my tolerance for talking to people I didn't know. I couldn't muster the courage to ask whether the rest of the food – which had been touching the black pudding – had been replaced. I drank my tea and we left. I breakfasted on gluten-free biscuits in the cabin later.

I returned from this holiday doubtful I'd ever be able to travel and eat safely away from home again. Unfortunately, our local restaurants performed no better. My first meal out after diagnosis was at a small ristorante in London with a good reputation for its gluten-free menu. The owner seemed unfazed when I explained I couldn't eat gluten. "No problem," he said. He often served a very famous diner who was also a coeliac. He was particularly fond of the gluten-free pasta. That sounded encouraging. A kitchen that knew its stuff. One bowl of Kamut pasta please.

The meal was tasty, but I began to feel bloated within a few minutes of leaving the restaurant. A quick Google search revealed kamut to be an ancient healthy grain, supposedly easy on the digestion. Sounded good. An ancient, healthy type of wheat. What? Bloody funny definition of gluten-free. "Awfully sorry," the owner said when we rang. He hadn't realised. Would we like a free meal by way of apology? But I'd had my fill of restaurants. I wondered what kind of pasta their famous guest would be served next time he visited.

After the pasta disaster, I tried to get my head around the changes I'd need to make to my eating habits and lifestyle. We'd just moved house. I had a toddler, no car and intermittent energy levels, so I didn't get out much beyond the garden gate. Once our daughter Helena was born, I had two children under four. Even my birding journal screeches to a halt in these early years of motherhood, my diaries filled instead with random jottings about the plants I was getting to know in the greenhouse and borders.

Initially, our new garden felt static, weighed down with so many shrubs, with nowhere to grow fruit trees, herbs, vegetables or perennial flowers. I hate waste, so I put an offer on Freecycle:

free plants, bring your own spade. A succession of local gardeners arrived over the next week, dug up the shrubs we didn't want and carted them off, each rehoming leaving more potential in its wake. Little by little, the garden I planned began to take shape.

I made the 9 metres by 13 metres space work hard for its keep, squeezing in a couple of raised vegetable beds and the smallest fruit cage I could find, as well as a flowerbed, shed and tiny spring garden with daffodils and snake's-head fritillaries. We kept the lawn for the kids to play on, but added a narrow border down the left-hand side for one of my dream kitchen garden additions: three espalier apple trees. Though I made room for a few shrubs and planted the narrow strip we shared with our next-door neighbours with Russian sage, globe thistles and lavender for pollinators, my main aim was to grow edibles. One of the incentives for moving had been to find a garden with more room for fruit and vegetables. Now we were here, I was determined to get the fruit trees in as soon as possible. Timing, I knew from bitter experience, was all-important. The plum tree in our old garden had produced its first decent crop of fruit the year we moved house. Weeks of gooseberry crumble and summer puddings had served only to whet my appetite for the ripening plums. We'd exchanged contracts and agreed on a completion date when it suddenly dawned on me that we'd made a terrible error with the schedule. We were due to move in early August. A couple of weeks before plumfection in the garden of the house we were leaving.

I was not sorry to say goodbye to our small shady plot, but I mourned the abandoned harvest for the rest of the summer. I wondered if the new tenants liked plums. Would they notice the bumper crop, realise what juicy delights hung in the tiny bed behind the garage? Perhaps the harvest I'd waited for years to come to fruition would be left to fall and rot. I contemplated scaling the fence at dusk, scrumping bag in hand. *Nip over, swipe any neglected plums and out again before anyone notices...* but I'm a law-abiding wimp at heart, so I settled instead for scouring nursery catalogues for fruit trees for our new garden.

My first choice was Opal, a plum–gage cross sometimes known as the early Victoria. Its sweet fruit remind me of the year I first tried Victoria plums in my friend Emma Pratt's front garden when I was ten; the same year we scared ourselves silly watching *Raiders of the Lost Ark* and ate so much deep-pan ham and pineapple pizza that I was sick. I never forgot the Elysian sweetness of those plums and I've detested pineapple with ham ever since.

After Opal, I had space for one more tree. In the end, I plumped for another link to my past. Like my grandpa, greengages are my favourite fruit. If I had once thought Victoria plums the food of the goddesses, they were knocked out of the celestial top spot when I ate my first greengage. I imagine Grandpa as a little boy in shorts in the 1920s, his wispy white hair still thick and blond, his mouth sticky from gorging on scrumped greengages in his Suffolk village: a honeyed hangover of a bygone age. And I love to grow plants with a local history, so I chose Cambridge Gage – a supersweet variety thought to have been raised from a seedling of Old Green Gage and first grown commercially at the beginning of the twentieth century by Chivers and Sons, fruit farmers and jam makers based in Histon, just north of Cambridge.

After the greengage, there was no more room in the back garden for standard trees, but there was a drab fence to cover, so trained fruit seemed the obvious choice. October saw us munching our way through Apple Day at Ryton Organic Gardens to see which varieties tickled our taste buds. We picked James Grieve, Egremont Russet and the dual-purpose cooker/eater Bountiful and, when we got back, I placed a bare-root order. I planted the young fruit trees that winter and trained them over the next few years as four-tiered espaliers – all apart from James, whose top right arm I accidentally cut off. He never forgave me. Eventually, a cordon Fiesta apple, a patio cherry and a Meech's Prolific quince filled every tree-sized space.

I work in the garden. I have visions of my children napping beside me in the pram. I know I spent hours outside as a baby, asleep. Even in the snow, Mum says, she'd wheel me out, snuggled in blankets. I might have been well wrapped, but some sleeping part of me must have known I was outside. My nose, perhaps. I wonder if that's why something settles inside me when I feel the breeze on my cheeks and hear the birds. I assume that outdoor naps will bring my children that same sense of inner peace. I'm quickly disabused of my naïve assumptions. My bairns turn out to be pickles, incapable of sleeping unless they're being pushed in the buggy or carried in a sling.

So I bring the playpen outside or they play on the slide or drive round the lawn in a red-and-yellow push-along toy car while I snatch a few moments to prick out seedlings, plant annuals or sow radishes in the raised beds. And while I work, we sing. Our whole life is a song. We have lyrics for every part of the day and, when we do something the toddler singing classes haven't predicted, I come up with new ditties or improvise extra verses. The kids 'help' me with the gardening. We lash beanpoles together and string up old sheets and blankets to make tents. Col films Helena's first wobbly steps across the lawn. On videos and photos, I'm invariably somewhere in the background, pottering about with trowel and trug. Watching the footage, I'm reminded of my early gardening days, when time (if you believe old photos) is measured via my succession of variously coloured wellington boots. Toddler-me sports yellow wellies that reach up to my pudgy knees. I carry a matching yellow bucket and gesture at the camera in a serious manner; perhaps I'm raising my hand to speak. A year or so later I'm wearing red wellies and a quilted blue anorak. I look completely at home squatting in the vegetable patch gathering sticks. Then comes the pond-dipping shot. I'm a little girl now: glossy black wellies, blue cotton trousers, a magnificent bowl haircut. Of all the heinous hairstyles I was subjected to as a child, this photograph is surely evidence of the worst offender. It swallows even my eyebrows. I like the wellies, the buckets and the sticks. I want all those for my kids. But I'll spare them the haircut.

Before I start planting up the vegetable beds, I set myself a couple of ground rules:

Rule No. 1: No growing vegetables I don't like. That won't help me fall in love with cooking and eating again. And that means you, runner beans. A pity really because the flowers have an undeniable beauty, especially bicoloured varieties like Painted Lady and the subtle apricot shades of Sunset, and, as climbers, they provide a substantial harvest in a small space. I fall off the wagon just the once and sow White Lady. I try so hard to make my peace with the pods, but to no avail. Unlike Nigel Slater, I cannot like the smell of freshly cut runner beans. While he imagines blending their fragrance with *l'odeur de* cut grass and sliced cucumber to create the essence of a British summer, I choke back memories of stringy fibrous balls that had to be swallowed.

Also, no swedes. And I have tried my best with this one. Roasted, boiled, sautéed, with garlic, ginger, bacon. I swear there is no agreeable way to cook a swede. Truth be told, my palate can't forgive them for infiltrating my mashed carrots all those years ago and turning the whole plateful into a bitter-tasting slush. Oh, and no broad beans either. Not that there are any bad childhood memories here, I just don't like them. Perhaps it's embarrassing as an advocate of growing your own to admit how many vegetables I dislike. But I can't see the point of growing stuff you hate. Apart from rainbow chard, of course. I'm a sucker for anything brightly or unusually coloured. I choose All Gold raspberries and a pink-fruited blueberry, sow Yellowstone and Purple Haze carrots, Hungarian Black chillies, Green Zebra, Golden Sunrise and Indigo Rose tomatoes, the latter ripening to blue-black except under the calyx, which can be lifted to reveal an alluring flash of red skin. The kids explore this rainbow of fruit and vegetables: sowing, picking, tasting, taking it all in. Sometimes I wonder when I'll get the call from nursery: "Hello Mrs Wilson. Hope you're well. We'd just like a word about your son's vision. He insists this morning that raspberries are yellow, tomatoes black and carrots purple. We think it advisable you get his eyes tested."

Rule No. 2: The garden will be a place to experiment with exciting new flavours. As I can no longer eat my way across the world by visiting the restaurants in town, I plan to grow my own ingredients for a range of cuisines. I start in Mexico with the cucamelon. This climbing plant in the squash family, also known as the mouse melon or Mexican sour gherkin, produces bite-size pale green fruits streaked with dark stripes and squiggles. Picked at just the right moment, these tiny taste-bombs deliver a burst of lime, watermelon and cucumber, but leave them to grow any bigger than olives and overnight they become rubbery and bland. I often meet gardeners who tell me they've grown cucamelons, only to decide they're not worth the hype.

"How big do you let them grow before you pick them?" I ask.

"About this big" – thumb and forefinger indicating the length of a small plum.

Size matters. Years later, in an effort to disseminate the 'eat 'em small' message, I write an article called 'Do My Cucamelons Look Big in This?' and hope, as a result, that readers all over the country will harvest teeny-weeny cucamelons and rejoice in their zesty glory.

While exploring Mexico's edible plants, I meet the tomatillo – a key ingredient of Mexican salsa verde. I fell in love with Tex-Mex and Mexican food while travelling round the US and, when I returned to England in autumn 1995, Chiquito in the Gateshead Metrocentre seemed the height of dining sophistication and adventure. I learned to cook burritos, fajitas, enchiladas, quesadillas, tacos, corn soup, and discovered a taste for Desperados – a French lager flavoured with agave spirit. But I've never come across the tomatillo before. Growing these tangy fruits that swell secretly, stickily inside papery husks until they burst through reawakens my interest in Mexican cuisine. We chop them into guacamoles and salsas, cook them in soups and stews. It becomes a challenge to find new ways to use tomatillos and every fresh recipe reminds me of the pleasures of cooking and eating.

Leaving Mexico, I journey 4,000 miles south-east to Chile where I find the fruit reputed to be Queen Victoria's favourite – the Chilean guava. I choose this relative of myrtle as a low, evergreen alternative to box hedging, which has recently discovered so many blighty, mothy ways to die. Chilean guava plays the part of a sober shrub with conviction, maintaining its low profile until early autumn when the tiny pink fruits can no longer contain themselves. While weeding old man's beard out of the gravel beds, I can smell the bawdy sweetness of toffeed strawberries stealing across the garden. The kids pick them as after-school snacks and persuade our neighbours to try them. Unlike blueberries, they retain their shape when cooked in cupcakes. Every mouthful reminds me why I love growing these special fruits.

I find it hard to set sail from the Americas. I'm obsessed with rootling about in the Andes, whose tuberous goodness knows no bounds. There's yacon, mashua and my favourite of all tubers: oca. I start with Helen's All Red oca and the promise of delicious lemony tubers come November or early December. Planted out after the last frost, the harvest is duly unearthed a few weeks before Christmas, glimpses of scarlet nuggets glistening in my otherwise sleepy winter garden. The colour is arresting, but why so small?

I find the answer to this question on the website of the Guild of Oca Breeders, which explains that this high-altitude Andean plant starts to form tubers only once the days become shorter in the autumn. This leaves oca too little time to grow to a substantial size before frosts hit. The guild is working on developing a long-day variety that will crop well in the northern hemisphere.

I find oca fascinating. Before I know it, I've volunteered for the Guild of Oca Breeders' citizen science project. The following spring, 13 unnamed varieties arrive in a slightly damp suspiciously shaped package. I grow them in pots and then transplant them into a bed in the allotment, protecting them from the local muntjac with copious netting and a good dollop of hope. Over the growing season, I note foliage colour, flowering periods, stem length, plant vigour and, finally, the size and weight of the crop. I participate in the trials for only a year but I continue to grow oca from the best of my starter tubers.

Before leaving the Andes, there's the small matter of an intriguing seedy present from a friend. "Try growing this," she says, with a grin. I plant the knobbly flat black seeds and they grow into rampant vines that attempt to throttle my windowsill seedlings. One gets a tendril around the neck of a plastic diplodocus and smothers it in a slo-mo hug. Achocha – one of many names for this aggressive creeper with aspirations of world domination – has curious fruits that resemble small prickly aliens, according to my kids. A friend calls them veghogs. They taste a little like mild green peppers when cooked and grow so prolifically that even the kids tire of achocha pizza long before the season is over.

From the Andes, I cross the Pacific Ocean and both the Philippine and South China Sea to Vietnam. All for a few leaves of perennial coriander. Regular coriander no sooner germinates in my garden than it's bolted and run to seed. Give Vietnamese coriander a moist, sunny spot and it will reward you through the summer with spicy leaves not dissimilar in taste to the annual herb. This is just the first of a series of plants that kick off my passion for Thai cooking. I add a range of chillies (one year I realise I've accidentally grown over 50 plants of 13 varieties in my desperately overcrowded greenhouse), garlic, Thai basil, lemongrass and makrut lime, and we dine on curries all summer long.

On the way home from Asia, I stop off in Liguria in north-west Italy to get to know the most phallic of crops: the tromboncino. The best thing about these giants, apart from their comedy value, is the long seedless neck like an overstretched butternut squash. The flesh is soft and sweet. Delicious in stir fries and courgette and chilli cornbread. Our most impressive specimen in the first year grows to a mighty 80 centimetres. Yet this is a mere stripling compared to the magnificent tromby grown by an astonished gardener in Nottingham from a seed he's been given as a present. It reaches a whopping 173 centimetres and is declared a European record at the Malvern Autumn Show. His response to growing this big boy makes me laugh. He's a meat and veg man, he says, and by that he means normal-looking veg. He doesn't intend to tuck into his monster tromboncino. Not for him the endless months of ratatouille, pickles and tromboncino cake. Instead, he plans to save the seed and attempt an even bigger one next year. It reminds me there are many ways to enjoy growing your own.

I love my garden. I've no doubt it plays a vital role in helping me live well with coeliac disease. If I hadn't grown my own fruit and vegetables, there'd have been little incentive to put aside the apathy that accompanied my dietary restrictions and get excited about cooking again. No reason to practise gluten-free shortcrust pastry for plum tarts and pies filled with home-grown beets, or sponge mix for Chilean guava cakes. We'd not have enjoyed the taste of fresh mint sauce, redcurrant cordial or tisanes sherbet-sweetened with lemon verbena. Several years after diagnosis I wrote about my garden in *Free-From Heaven* magazine as part of their series called 'My Free-From Life'. It was a significant moment – the first time I'd looked back and considered the impact of coeliac disease on my life. My piece began:

> Ever since I can remember I've wanted to be up at dawn, exploring the natural world at its most active, listening to the dawn chorus and engaging with the day in its infancy. In reality, most mornings I struggled to rise for work, or in the early days of motherhood, to soothe night-time toddler traumas.

I told the story of creating the first border at the stage when I could manage only a short time digging before retreating to bed for the rest of the day, and how the new diet improved my energy levels. I explained how raspberries and alpine strawberries inspired the kids to bake cupcakes and how the veg beds gave us the filling for gluten-free pasties. As the garden provided, we improvised. Cooking was dynamic, experimental and lots of fun. And though I wouldn't call myself a 'prolific gardener' and I swear I've never crimped a pasty in my life, it felt good to write about the way growing my own had helped me re-establish my relationship with food and the natural world.

But though gardening revived my appetite for life and connected me with the little patch of ground that I tended, it wasn't long before my roots began to feel pot-bound. Spiralling round and round the garden, searching for a way out, for something... bigger. Life seemed fenced in, tamed, though I wasn't sure how or why at the time. As I worked in the borders, I noticed self-seeders poking through the paving cracks, emerging from beneath the raised beds – red valerian, marjoram, lavender, old man's beard – but couldn't read them. I unearthed nubs of chalk as I dug holes for the fruit trees, but they were just lumps of rock. Red kites passed overhead, but they had no message for me yet. I couldn't see that my garden was sown with wild stories.

By the time my gluten-free diet awoke the energy within me, I was busy with the children. There was no opportunity to test my new strength by hiking in the mountains or along the coast, and it would never have occurred to me to do so. But as they grew, we ventured more often beyond the garden gate. I walked them to playgroup, to nursery, to school. Walking was both a necessity and a pleasant diversion from washing, feeding and cleaning: domestic tasks which were soothingly repetitive but which failed to occupy the relic fragments of a mind that early motherhood seemed to have taken hostage. And, as I walked, I began to notice.

The BFG

A series of dashes punctuate my days. Keeping time like an offbeat pendulum, I oscillate erratically, pitching up at the nursery gates just in time to kiss and release one bairn, then hurrying home with the other clasped against my chest in the sling. I bung in a wash and feed the baby. We play, cuddle, sing. Then rush back down the road for pickup, our two-and-a-half-hour morning over in what seems a mere 20 minutes. Life is hectic: mealtimes, naptimes, bath times, bedtimes... little time for anything else. Until one day, I start to read again.

After 12 years working full-time as an English teacher, while also completing a part-time MA in English literature, it's a relief to lay down my books now my bairns need me. I have no intention of returning to work at the end of maternity leave. Teaching requires so much physical and emotional energy – scarce resources at the best of times – that continuing my career seems incompatible with my role as a mother. The women in my family have always stayed at home to look after the children, so I assume the working chapter of my life is over and embark upon employment of a different kind, ploughing through piles of books passed on by family and friends, trying to digest unequivocal (but often contradictory) advice about parenting. But the self-assurance of the authors riles me, so I ditch the books, preferring instead to learn through trial and error. Turning to more inspiring fare, I read *Peepo!*, *Happy Dog, Sad Dog*, *Where's Spot?*, *Each, Peach, Pear, Plum*.

In the afternoons, while Helena naps, Jamie and I wander through the whimsical world of children's stories, reading and rereading our favourites: *Stick Man*, *Duck in the Truck*, *Meg and Mog*, *Cheese Hunt*. I read to him and he joins in, occasionally correcting my pronunciation when I use short northern vowels in words like 'grass' and 'bath'.

"You're saying it wrong, Mummy," he tells me solemnly. He's taught himself to read at three, it seems, with a giant alphabet jigsaw and countless episodes of *Alphablocks*. Watching his growing fascination with words and stories is one of the greatest joys of being a mum. By this point, I've almost forgotten I once spent my life immersed in literary fiction.

Then one evening, in a rare idle moment, I pick up Roger Deakin's 2007 nature classic *Wildwood*, a leaving present from a teaching colleague. Lured deep into the forest, I swiftly lose myself among the trees. One path leads to another and, over the next few years, my forays into nature books introduce me to new authors, ecologies and landscapes. I'm captivated by the eclectic mix of science, history, travel writing and personal narrative. I visit places I'll never see first-hand and cover more ground than my legs would ever manage. I meet people whose knowledge vivifies the world but from whom I would shy away in person. And I'm struck by how many of the journeys are predicated on active, purposeful engagement with the natural world. The writer, often male, strides out into the landscape in pursuit of a well-defined narrative goal, reminding me of my undergraduate dissertation on the hero quest – that archetypal journey covering long distances, spanning several counties, countries or continents with knowledge sought and gained before concluding with a return to the beginning.

I love the inspirational tenor of these stories, but I'm unnerved by their aspirational thrust. I measure the quality of my interactions with the natural world against the epic journey and the lone traveller, and find them wanting. More often than not, my encounters with the wild are incidental as I'm keeled by spring's first chiffchaff on the nursery run or lifted out of a melancholic half-slumber when house martins prospect the eaves above my window. In place of the quest narrative, my trips are episodic, repetitive, my trajectory drafted by a spirograph with the hiccups. I trace the same few paths in all lights and weathers, follow them in all moods and at wildly differing speeds. Am I gaining knowledge as I swing between nursery and home or from playgroup to the shops? Layering up slow intimacy in short, swift strokes, like Monet's series *Mornings on the Seine* that so fascinated me when I researched time and synchronicity for my MA? Every reiteration slightly offset, every subtle shift creating a more textured whole? Perhaps. My travels are certainly not ambitious or extraordinary in the ways that so many of my books describe. But neither are they without pattern or meaning. They are not diminished by their prepositional status, occurring on the way to (nursery), in between (naps), before or after (lunch). In fact, the fragmented nature of these journeys, punctuated by the routine tasks of washing, cleaning, watching television with the children or reading to them, cooking meals or getting them ready for bed, frees me to pursue a non-linear relationship with the local landscape and its history, one where tales are told by many voices, from many different times and places. As I become more familiar with my daily pathways and their stories, I wonder if life might be leading me in a new direction, towards an incidental counter-narrative.

Off on the nursery run: an expedition of 1,172 paces. The first of today's iterations. Six and a half minutes at a buggy-canter when we've had to nip back for mittens or a forgotten toy. Perhaps nine minutes if we've left enough time to linger, stretching to quarter of an hour when little legs trudge along beside me. At 315 paces, we cross the trainline over a footbridge that vaults a deep cleft in the chalk. In the late 1840s, when the Great Northern railway was on the move, the new line between London and York cut through Purwell Field – a large open field east of Hitchin – severing it in two. An arched brick bridge was constructed to connect nearby Purwell Mill with the town, allowing safe passage across the railway.

The first public train stopped at Hitchin in August 1850 and, one year later, a very special visitor arrived at the station. To the excitement of crowds of children lining the platform and, no doubt, the footbridge too, when the train stopped, Queen Victoria alighted. The monarch remained on the platform for only a matter of minutes to receive a basket of grapes and a bottle of lavender perfume prepared by local botanist and pharmacist William Ransom. William was part of a Quaker family of farmers, millers, bakers and landowners that had been based in the town for five generations. By 1851, he was running a flourishing pharmaceutical company cultivating and processing medicinal plants including lavender, for which Hitchin had long been renowned, so the perfume was an ideal symbol of the town's productivity and prosperity.

From their vantage point high on the bridge, not far from William Ransom's house on Benslow Hill, onlookers would have had excellent views of the Queen's train pulling into the station. Over the years, the long views up and down the track have made this a favoured place for young (and older) train spotters. In the mid-1970s, one Hitchin octogenarian recalled how it was a 'great joy to many youngsters, both boys and girls, and I think to their fathers too, who would run from one side of the bridge to the other as the smoke from the steam trains bellowed up'. So when I stop on the way back from nursery to peer through the railings with the kids, we're just the latest in a long line of local train spotters.

Crossing the bridge is the most unnerving part of our daily commute. Electrification of the line in the 1970s spelled the end of the much-loved brick footbridge, when Operation Live Wire required more clearance than its low-slung arch could provide. The Victorian bridge was blown up and replaced with a modern footbridge. So rather than feeling reassuringly solid bricks beneath our feet, we cross on precast concrete decking, supported by two concrete and two steel pillars, which bounces alarmingly when our footsteps fall in sync. The wobble in the bridge and my knees intensifies towards the middle. I grasp the children's hands tightly. They don't know I'm holding on as much for my sake as for theirs.

We often stop to wave to the engine drivers. While Jamie counts the trains with his endless endearing refrain "Just one more, Mummy", I walk my eyes along the cutting, noting how the chalk is exposed here and there. Now cloaked with ash, dogwood, field maple, self-sown apple trees and scrambling old man's beard, the bare chalk face would once have been far more extensive. When the cutting was excavated, the large cap of gravel on top of the hill was used to ballast the line for miles around. Great mounds of sand sifted out of the gravel were used by John Ransom, William Ransom's father, on his hilltop estate. The newly created cliffs, which rise 100 feet above the line, were quarried for chalk to supply the lime kilns belonging to William Ransom's older brother Alfred. Above the chalk layer, the bare faces of thick veins of sand were tunnelled and then inhabited in summer by a thriving colony of sand martins.

One summer's day in 1879, workmen on the line heard cries of alarm and distress coming from above. Looking up, they saw a stoat climbing one of the perpendicular cliff faces, slipping into the holes and dragging out sand martin chicks. I imagine the sooty forms of the adults sheering out from the cliff, flashing their white bellies. How they'd wheel above our heads. How we'd point and wonder, just a few steps from our front door. But the nearest breeding sand martins are over 12 miles away now, the colony in the railway cutting long gone. If it hadn't been for an opportunistic stoat over a century ago, I don't imagine anyone alive today would realise sand martins had ever been here at all.

Handwash Only
Wash Dark Colours Separately
Iron on Reverse

Back home, after the first nursery run of the day, I peg out the washing. A row of faded babygrows, flapping muslins, teeny socks and towelling nappies. Some of the more delicate garments that were given as gifts should no doubt be hand-washed, but I can't be doing with all that faff. They go in with Jamie's hand-me-downs and settle to companionable shades of grey. Once dry, they'll sit in a pile with the rest of the clean washing until I get round to sorting them – probably when I run out of nappies and set out on an emergency hunt. Clothes form these shifting piles all around the house, like mountain ranges thrown up by the unpredictable movement of tectonic plates. No sooner have I conquered one peak than another arises in a new location. Such proliferating heaps have one advantage: the higher they grow, the more weight presses on the garments at the bottom of the pile. I barely ever iron, but this way I can convince myself I'm making a strategic decision. I'm harnessing the power of gravity to flatten Col's work shirts in a process we call geological ironing.

Beyond the train bridge on the nursery run, we make for the snickets up Benslow Hill. Past old gardens, fenced-off railway verges and scrawny hedges. By 732 paces, we're walking beside the grounds of Pinehill Hospital. Built in 1908 as a convalescent home for patients of the German Hospital in London, it accommodated both wounded British soldiers and German POWs during the First World War. Now filled with shrubs and mature trees, the large garden once supplied both Pinehill and the London German Hospital with fruit and vegetables. Between the wars, the hospital matron, a Lutheran sister from the Bodelschwingh Epilepsy Centre in Germany, arranged for a wood to be planted in a neighbouring field with young trees imported from her homeland. The woodland was described in later years as looking like a 'bit of Germany... transported to this German colony at Hitchin'. Although many of the trees were later felled by the council, some of the pines around the field edge were left standing and have since developed into impressive specimens. I wonder how many patients over the decades have taken comfort from the wooded view beyond the grounds.

Looking up at the trees, I think back to my time in Pinehill Hospital. Having been referred to the coeliac clinic for an endoscopy, I have hazy memories of playing a surreal game of tag in a ground-floor room without a view, edging round the examining table away from the doctor as he tried to persuade me to lie down. I think I'd refused sedation – the thought of drowsy compliance terrified me – and I was halfway out of the door before Col was called in to calm me down. Later that day, I too looked out at the pines while recovering in an upstairs room. I remember the huge sense of relief once I could see nature's own tranquillisers. When I was sent for a second endoscopy two years later at the NHS hospital in Stevenage, a site not renowned for its extensive treescapes, I agreed to take the sedative.

1.45 **Something Special** *Justin and his friends are off to an exciting place to meet some British wildlife.*

2.05 **Mr Bloom's Nursery** *A group of Scouts make a huge pile of mashed potatoes at Mr Bloom's festival in Kilmarnock.*

2.30 **Show Me Show Me** *There is a vegetable show going on and Teddington has brought a big leafy cabbage.*

Morning pickup and lunch over, it's time for a CBeebies break. Our favourite programmes include *Chuggington*, *Octonauts* and *In the Night Garden*. Jamie is obsessed with building train tracks. He spends hours sliding along the floor, his cheek pressed against the carpet, choo-choo-ing wooden trains over level crossings and precariously balanced bridges. We all enjoy watching *Octonauts* and learn so much, but I have mixed feelings that the kids are more familiar with blobfish, coelacanths and immortal jellyfish than they are with hedgehogs or small tortoiseshell butterflies. Helena loves to sing and dance along with Upsy Daisy, Igglepiggle and the Tombliboos from *In the Night Garden*. She particularly likes performing the Tombliboos' song, complete with actions, ending with her arms spread wide – Pa-Dah! When Jamie was a toddler, he replaced the childlike phonetics of Tombliboo Unn, Ooo and Eee with "Tombliboo One", "Tombliboo Two" – so far, so good – and "Tombliboo Carrot" – I'm sorry, what? Now Helena takes her brother's Dadaist word game a step further as she attempts to name the *In the Night Garden* characters. She manages "Piggle" and "Daisy", then looks at the Tombliboos and says, quite clearly, "Bumhole". She smiles, very pleased with herself. We can't quite believe our ears. Perhaps her mispronunciation is the result of confusing the consonants in this trisyllabic word. Or perhaps our 18-month-old daughter is, like us, simply disturbed by the frequency with which the comedy trio lose their trousers.

Opposite the Pinehill Hospital, on the other side of the lane, a small front garden skirts the edge of the chalk cliffs. An abundance of ferns, spring bulbs, cottage garden perennials and alpines surround a central circular depression, rather like a miniature amphitheatre. Roses twine enthusiastically around the bungalow door. The chaotic planting intrigues and charms me every time I pass. I often see an older lady out and about, sometimes kneeling in the borders, head down, busy among the plants. I imagine her years of care have shaped this spirit-lifting garden.

Then one day, on our way to nursery, we notice building work. It seems the gardener and her bungalow have gone. Gone too her quirky, life-affirming garden. In its place, earth and rubble, then a new build with block-paved drive, garage and beech hedge. I feel wistful that the cherished garden is no more. I mention my sense of loss to a friend and she recollects her pleasure at the exuberant planting. Even now, she tells me, she sees the old patterns beneath the new. The collective nature of this memory pleases me, and I wonder how many other locals are reminded of the old garden as they pass by on their daily walks.

One autumn morning a couple of years later, a snapdragon startles me through the chain-link fence on the edge of this once-upon-a-time garden. Its cerise flowers are doubly surprising –

out of time and out of place – the lowest trumpets opening only now in mid-November while all around leaves drift down or hang with marcescent tenacity on the young beech hedge. Along with a couple of wilful scillas that still pop up in spring and a few small patches of cyclamen, this snapdragon is a botanical reminder of the garden's colourful history. I find it an apt anachronism. For me, snapdragons have long been symbolic of the past. Memories of long golden days outside with my dad, watching him perform that sudden transformation, turning an innocent flower into a mythic beast. How many of us remember our sense of wonder when the gentle pressure of thumb and forefinger made those hinged mouths yawn, the clustered dragonheads drawing us down to squeeze, peer and dream?

These days I grow snapdragons to connect my past with my children's present, watching them pinch and grin, much as I did. Like the lone chain-link survivor, my plants often self-seed and, though the resulting seedlings don't flower until late, some persist through our increasingly mild winters. It is, perhaps, fitting that the dragon's flowers are arranged facing outwards in different directions. They look back over our childhoods and the landscape's past while also pointing to the future. But though their post-aestival blooms cheer the eye on a dank November morning, I suspect they owe their success to our warming climate, and that makes their late flowering a bittersweet pleasure.

Ingredients: 2 ripe eating apples peeled, cored and chopped, 5 tablespoons of water or apple juice.
Method: Place the prepared apples in a pan with water or apple juice and cover. Cook on a low heat until soft, adding more water if apples start to stick. Leave to cool. Blend in a food processor until smooth. Freeze in ice-cube trays.

Back at home, I'm making lunch. It's that time again. Anything that stays still in my kitchen for more than a minute gets puréed. The colour of the purée determines how far from the walls I place seat and baby when feeding commences – innocuous pastes (apple, pear, baby rice) need only a restricted hazard zone with little protective equipment; the more vibrant purées (carrot, pea, blueberry) require comprehensive safety gear and a remote spot at the very centre of the kitchen. Weaning explosions aside, I find the process of puréeing an exceedingly comforting one. I remember how my mum brought me tomato soup and cheese on toast when I was ill, and Granny always had a pan of apples stewing, usually mixed with elderberries or blackberries. I was transfixed by the rich colours, wrapped in the heady smells of these homely concoctions. I hope my children will have similar memories. Nurturing begins here, I think. In the kitchen. Good food prepared with love.

Just over the crest of Benslow Hill, at 840 paces, a behemoth marks time behind a garden wall. It's easy to pass by without noticing if you're ploughing on, head down, intent upon your feet and your destination. But that's not how children walk. For them every flowerbed, every wall and pavement crack, offers tempting passage into magical worlds. So when we reach this special spot, we uncouple our necks and swing our heads back, eyes popping to the sky. The monster we're admiring looks completely out of place in this otherwise unexceptional front garden, like a giant's leg extruded from the clouds, a mythic flank flung far out of time and place. The bark of this giant sequoia is ridged and ruddy, thick and spongy, the vast trunk shooting skywards for 70 feet or more, entirely dominating the surrounding houses. Shaggy foliage spirals down from the apex like a helter-skelter, offering swift escape from the cloud-lands above. Around the foot of the tree, the ground swells as roots tussle with earth. How wonderful it would be to greet this Big Friendly Giant, skin to trunk in a three-person hug, but it is out of bounds in a private garden, so we must make friends from afar. Instead, getting to know this colossus requires a journey across the ocean to distant lands, travelling back through centuries, then millennia, for it seems we really have met a giant descended from myth and legend.

Our first stop is in the grounds of Fairfield House at the top of Benslow Hill, just across the road from where we now stand, in 1887. William Millard is working in the potting shed. He looks down at the handful of unfamiliar seeds he's just been given, each a dark-brown central pillar with papery wings. He sows them immediately and nurtures the emerging seedlings. Over the next year, he pots them on, places them under handlights out of doors, then transplants the saplings into a nursery bed where he protects them through harsh winters with mats and straw. In the autumn of 1901, he lifts and plants his unusual charges around the grounds of Fairfield House, where he works as a gardener to William Ransom. The 14-year-old saplings thrive, except where they have been planted too close to elm trees, whose hungry roots devour the water and manure before their young neighbours have a chance to get established.

William Millard's extraordinary teenagers are members of the largest tree species by volume on earth. They originate from the western slopes of the Sierra Nevada mountains in California and have been known over the years by many names, including giant sequoia, Wellingtonia (so called by the British in the Victorian period to the outrage of the Americans), *Sequoiadendron giganteum* or, simply, Big Trees. Introduced into the UK in the early 1850s, these colossal conifers quickly became popular in horticultural circles. Within a few years, young sequoias had been planted on many estates across the country. But while the Victorian fashion for cultivating giants was taking off in British gardens, their future in California seemed anything but secure.

European Americans first recorded and shared the location of the giant sequoia groves – which local Native Americans had known about for centuries – in 1852. Within a year, the first giant had been felled: a 1,244-year-old named the Discovery, or Mammoth, Tree. A second tree – Mother of the Forest, so called for her elegant shape and two protuberances resembling breasts – was stripped of her bark to a height of 116 feet just one year later. Bark from the girdled mother was sent to be displayed in Crystal Palace, no doubt encouraging the craze among wealthy Victorians for planting these trophy trees. Some keen botanists, like Hitchin's William Ransom, even travelled to California and collected their own seed. William's trip to the Sierra Nevada sequoia groves, where the stump of the Mammoth Tree was now being used as a dance floor, gave him the opportunity to see these giants in their natural habitat and collect cones so he could propagate his own trees. An extraordinary lithograph from 1862 shows a party of 32 people dancing on the Mammoth stump, which measured a gigantic 96 feet in circumference. It took five men 22 days to fell the tree. In the image, onlookers watch the dancing from horseback; one man even stands triumphantly on a platform atop a horizontal section of trunk, reached by a wooden ladder on which more people sit watching.

History doesn't record whether William Ransom danced a cotillion on the Mammoth Tree but, during his expedition in 1887, he visited two other ancient sequoias: the Grizzly Giant and the Wawona Tree. He was interested in the trees' dimensions and recorded the circumference of the Grizzly Giant – the oldest (at 2,995 years) and second largest tree in Mariposa Grove – at 93 feet near the ground. On visiting the Wawona Tree (a younger relative of the Grizzly Giant, at around 2,100 years old and a mere 90 feet in circumference), it seems likely he would have taken his turn on the stagecoach that rode through the famous Wawona Tree tunnel. This unfortunate tree was the second of several sequoias to have tunnels cut through their trunks. Perhaps, as a botanist, William might have disapproved of this practice, lamenting the internal injuries that a hole 7 feet wide, 9 feet high and 26 feet long would have caused the venerable sequoia. Whatever his views on felling, bark-stripping and tunnelling, he collected cones from the Grizzly Giant and Wawona Tree and brought his precious cargo back to Hitchin, entrusting the seeds to the care of his gardener.

As members of one of the world's fastest-growing conifer species, William Millard's young sequoias would have shot up. In their first decade, they may have grown up to 20 feet and, by the time he died in 1919, they could have reached an impressive 40 feet in height. Nothing else in his gardening experience would have prepared him for the vigour of these strapping saplings. Did he look up in astonishment, as Jack did when his beanstalk disappeared into the clouds, as we do now, and wonder if his precocious sequoias would one day tempt local children up to enchanted lands in the sky?

Now, more than a century after William planted out his saplings, the BFG on Benslow Hill towers over nearby ash, horse chestnut and pine. I can't understand why so many people walk past every day without raising their heads to wonder at the astonishing height of this youngster. For despite its grand name and distinguished heritage, compared to its 3,000-year-old Californian cousins our sequoia is a mere sapling. If it were measured against an oak tree with a lifespan of 600 years, it would be in its mid-20s. In human terms, it would be a similar age to Jamie and his nursery friends. And, with over 100 feet still to grow over the next three millennia before it approaches the heady heights of its putative parents, this Big Tree is only going to get bigger.

That's not my polar bear. Its nose is too squashy.
That's not my polar bear. Its paws are too bumpy.
That's my polar bear. Its tummy is so fluffy.

I rarely get time to tidy anything between nursery trips. Today, the lounge floor is strewn with *That's Not My* books, passed on by a friend. My favourite is *That's Not My Polar Bear*. The kids love to turn the pages and stroke bobbly noses, fuzzy ears and bumpy paws. Is this your monster? Your teddy? Your pirate? At night, Col and I make up our own versions:

That's not my mummy. Her energy levels are too high.
That's not my daddy. His temper is too even.
That's not my house. The floor is visible.

I love the way picture books bring stories alive, every repetition embedding characters and events deeper in our shared family experience. Together we decide why the unsuitable animals sent to us in *Dear Zoo* must, unfortunately, be sent back; we lick our lips at The Very Hungry Caterpillar's feast, then sympathise with its self-induced stomach ache; we set off on a bear hunt, squelching through Helena's favourite, the thick *oooozy* mud; we hide in the shed from Zachary Quack with Hairy Maclary from Donaldson's Dairy; and we lie down in the dark with Big Nutbrown Hare, listening as he tells us he loves us right up to the moon... and back.

I think about all the animal stories, from the earliest board books full of baby creatures and bird noises to older favourites such as *The Owl Who Was Afraid of the Dark* and the woodland wildlife scared away by the mouse with his tall tales of the Gruffalo. I think about how I've decorated the children's rooms – Jamie's underwater cavern where he swims with starfish and whales and turtles, Helena's parrot-, butterfly- and monkey-filled jungle paradise – about the false comfort we derive as parents from surrounding our kids with animals, while continuing to disregard and despoil the natural world upon which these creatures, and our own lives, depend. I wonder if, by the time my children's bairns start to read, polar bears, parrots and turtles will exist only in their stories alongside unicorns and dragons:

> That's not my polar bear. Its food source is too plentiful.
> That's not my polar bear. Its habitat is too stable.
> That's my polar bear. Its sea ice has all melted.

Back on Benslow Hill, in the silvery moonlight of the witching hour, the Big Friendly Giant sequoia is on the move. It steps lightly between the houses, blowing arboreal dreams through first floor windows. What stories will it share tonight? Perhaps local sleepers will travel 200 million years back in time to the birth of the sequoias in the humid Jurassic forests: luxuriant, green-hearted with ginkgoes, cycads and conifers. Or they might find themselves on the western slopes of the Sierra Nevada mountains on a clear May evening in 1903, where, at the foot of the Grizzly Giant, two men are turning in for the night. One, a stocky fellow with pince-nez and a walrus moustache, nestles deep into a pile of thin woollen army blankets; the other wraps himself in a piece of cloth and lies down beside his companion. The trunks of the sequoias rise around them like vast columns in a mighty cathedral and, from the darkening aisles, hermit thrushes sing melodious psalms.

It is the first evening of John Muir and Theodore Roosevelt's three-day camping expedition in Yosemite, a trip that Roosevelt requested and Muir welcomed as he has an agenda of his own to raise with the President – the protection of the forests and a species he affectionately calls the 'Big Tree'. The Scots-born polymath, naturalist, writer and ecological thinker first travelled through the Sierra Nevada mountains in the spring of 1868, at the age of 30. Over the next few years, Muir worked in Yosemite as a sheep-herder and in a saw mill, and began to write articles about conserving the natural environment. His ideas helped influence the US Congress decision to establish both Yosemite and Sequoia National Park in 1890, and the Sierra Club, which Muir co-founded in 1892, was instrumental in promoting conservation in the region.

No doubt as Muir and Roosevelt sat drinking coffee beneath the Grizzly Giant earlier that May evening, their conversation would have revolved around how to protect the forests and their Big Trees, which Muir considered 'king of all the conifers in the world'. At the end of the expedition, the two men parted on good terms, Roosevelt noting later that Muir talked even better than he wrote. Within three years, Yosemite Valley and Mariposa Grove would be included in the Yosemite National Park and, during his presidency, Roosevelt would establish 230 million acres of public lands, 150 million acres of which would be set aside as national forests. 'Any fool can destroy trees,' Muir wrote. But it took forward-thinking conservationists and politicians, like Muir and Roosevelt, working together to save the giants from extinction.

Twinkle, twinkle, little star,
How I wonder what you are!
Up above the world so high,
Like a diamond in the sky.

Singing lullabies to the children is a relaxing ritual for the whole family. Every evening, we sing 'Twinkle, Twinkle' to Helena and 'Lullaby, Lullaby, Going Upstairs to Bed Now' to Jamie. By the time we check on them before we go off to bed, they are usually warm, tousle-haired, sleeping deeply. Each with their own reassuringly familiar night-time scent. Jamie's bedroom smells of fresh sawdust, as if his duvet harbours a sleeping hamster. Helena is all musk and rose petals. I breathe in their essences, slowly, then find my own bed. Another long day closes.

For some unlucky souls, however, this evening's slumbers may well be a less congenial affair. As generations of children know, the Big Friendly Giant delivers only good dreams – winksquifflers or golden phizzwizards – unless a well-chosen bad dream might alert the sleeper to impending tragedy or they simply deserve a trogglehumping nightmare. So the Queen of England dreams of children being snatched out of their beds by ravenous giants, and Fleshlumpeater, the biggest and horriblest of all the giants, is tormented in his sleep by Jack the Giant-Killer. Perhaps, as an eleventh-hour warning, the Benslow BFG might spirit some dreamers to Mariposa Grove in 2022, at the hot end of one of the hottest of all Julys. At the base of the Grizzly Giant, where Roosevelt and Muir lay down to sleep over a century earlier, a sprinkler system has been installed to ensure the base of the trunk remains moist and thus more fire-resistant. Wildfires have been raging in the region all month, burning an area of nearly 5,000 acres, threatening to destroy the sequoias of Mariposa Grove and the nearby community of Wawona.

Fire has always been a key part of the giant sequoias' life cycle. Lightning is a regular cause of fire across the groves, and the resultant low intensity burns help dry out mature cones high in the canopy, which then release their seeds. Fire-stripped soil provides bare patches for germination, ash acts as a fertiliser, and the emerging saplings benefit from improved light levels in the newly cleared understorey. Native Americans had long understood the vital role of natural fires in maintaining forest ecosystems, but European American settlers saw only a destructive force, which they believed threatened the survival of the groves. For a century from the 1860s onwards, fires were prevented and, consequently, a dense layer of trees, shrubs and dead wood built up, creating a perfect tinderbox. Despite the sequoia's fire-resistant layer of spongy bark, and branches that grow high enough in mature trees to escape most natural fires, these ancient adaptations give them little protection against the ferocity of the new megafires.

It's ironic that the very natural force that facilitates reproduction is one of the main factors threatening the future of the sequoias. In the six years leading up to the Washburn Fire near Mariposa Grove in 2022, wildfires ripped through large areas full of accumulated fuel after years of drought and beetle damage. During this time, more than 85 per cent of all the giant sequoia grove area was burned, as opposed to only a quarter in the entire preceding century. The Castle Fire in 2020 raged through the King Canyon National Park and the Sequoia National Forest from mid-August until December, killing between 10 and 14 per cent of the world's oldest and largest sequoias (sometimes referred to as monarch sequoias). The following year, the Windy Fire destroyed another 5 per cent. Some experts fear these gentle giants might be completely eradicated in the wild, leaving only the younger, smaller trees. The figures associated with this loss would be mind-boggling. Tens of thousands of monarchs, many of which are thousands of years old, each with a lineage that stretches back hundreds of millions of years. Destroyed by a species with whom they have shared the planet for only 300,000 years, one that measures its lifespan in decades rather than millennia. Giant sequoias might grow 50 times as tall and live 50 times as long as humans, but their superior height and longevity count for little when climate change-induced wildfires sweep through the groves. The US National Parks Service and the US Forest Service are trying to remedy more than a century of fire suppression by restoring the sequoia groves and removing dead trees. The race is now on to reduce fuels in the remaining unprotected groves before the next megafires; otherwise we risk our generation supplanting Jack as the most infamous of all giant-killers.

The seeds of these stories are sown as I hurry back and forth, the details garnered from repeated observation, natural history journals, maps, museum archives and talking to local folk. I am fascinated by the lives of those who studied the wildlife and landscape in previous centuries. Some days I'd not be surprised to come across William Ransom in the snickets, crouched down, studying some plant or other by the side of the path. As I walk to nursery or the shops and learn about the history of the landscape, the boundaries between fact and fiction, observation and imagination, past and present become so porous, they all but dissolve. Though my stories are rooted in the local, they transport me through time and space without the need to stray more than a few hundred paces from my own front door.

And, all this while, during all of these short trips, I don't sink down by the wayside because I can't walk any further. I no longer regularly kneel at the bottom of the stairs, staring up the unscalable ascent. On a gluten-free diet, I'm a physically stronger version of myself. But, deep down, I know my energy levels still aren't normal. Travelling in dreams and imagination is sometimes as much as I can manage. Every few months, in the blur of life with small kids, I lose a week or two to illness and severe fatigue, sometimes more, my bed-realmed days, as always, excised from short-term memory the instant I recover. There are periods of anxiety and depression too, weeks where I haunt the house in a heavy-hearted daze.

But I have decided on my story and I stick to it. I tell friends how lucky I am to get my diagnosis. Not many people enter their late 30s with more energy than they've had since their teens. I tell them long-term fatigue is a thing of the past, and I believe it too. I convince myself I have left the woman I despise – the woman who gets ill – behind me. As she impinges on my freedom less, I ignore her more easily. I construct the fiction I think friends and family want to hear: a cheerful account of illness, diagnosis and recovery. A 15-year quest, fulfilled. I might be considering a counter-narrative, but I have no intention of giving it an unhappy ending.

Snickets

Eight years after I went on maternity leave with my eldest, I kissed my youngest and waved her into reception for her first day at school. She was ready for a new adventure and we were confident she would thrive. Back at home, without the routine of her day to structure mine, I felt unmoored. Most of my local friends still had preschool children, so they continued to meet up at playgroup and music classes. But my life had moved on. I wondered where it was taking me.

While the children were at school, I busied myself with chores and gardening, enrolled on a garden design diploma one day a week at Regent's Park and walked the local paths around town, enjoying the opportunity to dawdle and daydream. I spent hours getting to know the plants I met along the way, learning about their botany and history. I remembered how, as a child, I'd found back alleys unnerving, especially those lined with crumbling walls or towering evergreen hedges. But they were magical portals too – transporting you from place to place like the secret passages in Cluedo. You could vanish in one street and materialise three streets down; sidle into the park via the back route; take a shortcut to town along footpaths that slipped quietly between the houses.

In the North West, we called these pathways 'snickets', one of many regional terms that include Cornwall's opes, Norfolk's lokes, Birmingham's gullies and Scotland's pends. In different areas of the UK, we might follow the jigger or jog up the shut; cut through ginnel, vennel or gitty; hurry into the wynd; disappear down twitten or twitchell; gain the tenfoot or leg it along the lonnin. We enter these marginal spaces via old words that twist the mouth and lead the mind. Sometimes they had less salubrious meanings too. Liverpool's jiggers could refer to prison cells and illegal distilleries, and snickets was a slang term for outsiders: misers, saucy lasses, insolent women or naughty children – historically maligned and marginalised figures, their unsavoury characteristics hidden by society until they could be effaced or transformed. Just so with our back passages, our dog-shit alleys: unremarkable places of lurking subversion, danger and dirt.

Our daily pursuit of throughways and shortcuts favours destination over journey. Snickets are paths with the end, often quite literally, in sight. Even the ubiquitous 'alley' derives from the Old French *aler*: to go, foregrounding movement over place. When I stop en route to take a photograph of my favourite patch of white violets or identify a new plant, pedestrians pass me by without pausing. Crouched in the verge, barely a metre from the path, I am so far off the beaten track that my presence hardly registers. At times like this, I wonder where our antipathy to lingering comes from. Why such unwillingness to surrender our sense of direction and purpose, if only for a moment? The pace of modern life certainly leaves little space for interludes, but perhaps there is an element of fear too. Of faltering and falling into the unknown. Of waking to a fecund reality where wild couples with cultivated, public enters private, and past roots in present while furtively setting seed for the future.

But I enjoy my encounters with natural history and the history of the natural in these transitional spaces. Exploring narrow alleyways where courtyard ornamentals escape through wall crevices to colonise the pavement edges, slipping through concealed entrances that open only for those who hide and seek, roaming the broad beech paths that edge the town and emerge from the outermost estates into rural rides of generous scope and dappled sunspots. When my movements are constrained by timetables and energy levels, snickets are my escape into the wild. Within their narrow confines, like the mysterious Cole Hawlings in *The Box of Delights*, I can go small or swift and, best of all, I can travel in time.

Walking through Hitchin's snickets feels like exploring the footnotes of local history. Many of the paths are old ways, repositories of long-forgotten stories. Overlaying a conjectural map of the nine open fields surrounding Hitchin around the beginning of the sixteenth century onto Google Earth reveals surprisingly few changes to the pathways over the past five centuries. Many of the routes persist today due to the long continuity of the open field system hereabouts. Some areas around Hitchin even remained unenclosed into the early twentieth century, far longer than in many towns and villages, where enclosures in the eighteenth and nineteenth centuries radically altered the structure and politics of the landscape.

Between 1766 and 1832, the common fields of 22 parishes within 10 miles of Hitchin were enclosed. Similarly, my shepherding ancestors 50 miles north in Helpston, Northamptonshire, lived through enclosure in the early nineteenth century. They rented rooms in the same house as the poet John Clare during this period. My great-great-great-great-grandfather worked in the field gangs during enclosure; his name is listed in the same labour accounts as Clare. Both he and the poet, along with many other villagers, earned money fencing and hedging the fields while also suffering the dispossession that resulted from the loss of common land.

As people were denied access to places they had relied on for foraging, grazing livestock, fuel gathering and communal festivities for generations, their stories were marginalised, their lives edited out of the heart of the landscape. Over the centuries, agriculture and development consumed the remaining margins until, in many places, the old tracks and tales became inaccessible, unreadable, functionally extinct.

Most of my local journeys take place within the area that used to be Purwell Field, one of Hitchin's largest open fields. In 1883, Frederic Seebohm, the economic historian and banker who lived in the town from 1855 to his death in 1912, published *The English Village Community*. In this seminal book, Frederic examined the field system, using his local area as a case study. He noted there were 289 strips in Purwell Field around 1770, owned by 48 individuals. This made it impractical to obtain agreement for enclosure, which required consent of the owners of 75 per cent of the land by value. By 1816, the 11 largest landowners in the town owned around 66 per cent of the fields, not enough to secure an enclosure act, and not all landowners were in favour of enclosure. Consequently, much of Purwell Field remained open into the early twentieth century. As the area around my house was gradually developed, small estates were fitted within the existing furlong framework, and ancient field paths were surrounded by houses, the old ways reborn as suburban snickets.

The maps in Frederic Seebohm's book show a network of field strips and access paths criss-crossing Purwell Field. He describes the 'little narrow strips' on a tithe map from around 1816 as 'almost the features of a spider's web' separated by 'green balks of unploughed turf', and explains that 'the whole arable area of an unenclosed township was usually divided up by turf balks into as many thousands of these strips as its limits would contain'. The strips were grouped into furlongs, often called 'shots' or 'shotts' in Hertfordshire. Each furlong had a common field way alongside it that gave access to the strips, or a headland within the furlong boundary for the strip owners to walk to their land and turn their ploughs. People owned intermixed strips in different furlongs scattered across the common field, and often across several fields. This created a community of owners who sowed, ploughed and left their strips fallow in conjunction with each other.

The small section of Purwell Field that Frederic Seebohm chose to demonstrate strip and furlong arrangements includes the area around my house. The field path along Long Shadwell Shot's headland now forms an unmarked snicket where I found an abandoned wasps' nest last autumn, fallen from a bramble patch. Over the road, the line of the old field way becomes Benslow Path and crosses the railway, leading between houses (on what was once Benchley Hill Shot) and a school (on what was Beggarly Shot). As the snicket turns left, cutting the corner as it has for centuries, it meets a narrow rectangular plot of three houses which looks like an afterthought backing onto a larger estate. On Frederic's map, this strip marks out the headland for Wymondley Highway Shot. Looking over the hedge today, I see only paving and houses, but for hundreds of years the headland would have given locals access to their field strips and would have been the last strip to be ploughed. Where parents now stand chatting, waiting for their kids to come out of school, centuries of conversations have taken place. Different topics, different times, but the same gathering of local people.

Some furlong names give an insight into the nature of the land itself. Short Shadwell Shot (the shallow springs), Riddy Shot (the small stream) and, on the margins of Purwell Field, Ninesprings and Rushmead (the meadow where the rushes grow) highlight the prevalence of upwellings from the chalk bedrock, forming pools, brooks and marshy areas. Other furlongs read like a found poem:

Welshmans Croft, Cow Common Lammas, Nettle Dell
Sparrow Bush Shot, Hag Dell Shot, Duck Land
Manley Highway Shot, Furson Hedges
Purwell Grove, Moor Mead Bottom, Crow Furlong

These names send me back through the centuries, their references to wildlife, livestock, people and place hinting at old lives and stories. Landscape history is so often forgotten, but remembering is important, even if all that remains of meads, hedges, bushes and animals are their names. They act as signposts indicating where we've come from and, more evocatively – disturbingly – where we're going.

Beggarly Shot was one of the larger furlongs in Purwell Field. Despite its derogatory name, which referred to its inferior soil quality, the infertile, chalky ground was ideal for growing lavender. By the 1860s, William Ransom was growing 40 acres of this tough, aromatic plant around Hitchin, some of it in or around Beggarly Shot. Lavender already had a long history in the town. Supposedly grown here since the sixteenth century, it began to be cultivated as a commercial crop from the early 1800s. By the late nineteenth century, Hitchin was one of the three principal centres for lavender production in the UK. In the summer of 1863, chemist Charles W. Quin was invited on a tour of William Ransom's physic farm. He describes one of many fields the two men visited, where the lavender was in full bloom. Quin wrote:

> it would take the pen of a Ruskin to give our readers any idea of the beauty of the sight. The long spikes of purple flowers waving backwards and forwards in the gentle wind, interspersed with the delicate greenish-grey of the plants themselves, and patches of golden brown soil showing between them now and then, make up a picture worthy of the pencil of our great colourists.

I don't need John Ruskin or the great colourists to imagine Hitchin's fields awash with purple. Since 2000, the Hunter family have revived this local tradition, growing lavender at Cadwell Farm just north of the town. We visited often when the children were younger. While they picked lavender and played in the gardens, I'd wander the trial fields, exploring the different growth habits, scents and colours of the 60 varieties on show.

Over the years, I have bought many lavender plants for my garden, including Twickel Purple, Edelweiss, Munstead and Blue Ice. They self-seed in the gravel and put down roots in the paths, as if they are trying to tell me this dry, chalky land is part of their story – and they of its.

As well as lavender, William cultivated deadly nightshade, along with squirting cucumber, henbane, foxglove, aconite, peppermint and poppy. These species were grown as ingredients for his galenical, or plant-based, preparations, which included remedies for afflictions of the eyes, whooping cough and acute rheumatism. Although William's crops were destined for medicinal use, there were risks associated with living near his fields. Quin's account of the squirting cucumber explains that 'the force with which the seeds are driven out is so great, that Mr Ransom frequently finds the country children who gather the cucumbers crying bitterly from the force of the blow'. Surrounded by henbane, aconite and deadly nightshade, local youngsters were no doubt taught at a young age not to pick or eat plants.

Nearly a century later, William Ransom & Son was cultivating around 35 acres of deadly nightshade. Through much of the twentieth century local school children were warned about the dangers of eating the glossy purple berries, as by this point the plant had escaped into the verges and surrounding waste ground. Unlike concerned parents and teachers, a pair of redstarts that nested and reared young for three consecutive years above the evaporating pans in the Ransom factory didn't seem bothered by the toxic properties of deadly nightshade.

Cultivation stopped in the mid-twentieth century but deadly nightshade left its mark on the land. Rogue self-seeded plants would appear between the rows of roses in the nursery at the top of Benslow Hill, on land which once belonged to William Ransom. Even now, the occasional plant pops up in nearby gardens and I've found them along the snicket that runs up through the estate where the nursery used to be. Although deadly nightshade grows wild in the UK, the *Flora of Hertfordshire* suggests occurrences of the plant near Hitchin are likely to be escapes from past cultivation. Their presence reminds me of the unseen history in the margins. When I go on the school run or walk down to town, seed-memories lie beneath my feet, waiting for the opportunity to return and re-establish their roots in the chalk.

Another old path reborn as a suburban snicket, Riddy Lane, leads away from the town if you are seeking space and solitude in the fields, as I often am. More importantly, for labourers returning from a day harvesting mangelwurzels or cabbages two centuries ago, it would have stretched back towards habitation and their evening meal. Starting near Ippollitts Brook on the south side of Hitchin, Riddy Lane now runs between two rows of fence-lined back gardens but, for at least half a millennium, until the early twentieth century, it was the main route across this part of Purwell Field. 'Riddy' is a local word derived from the Old English *rith* or *rithig*, meaning a small stream or intermittent rill. In Hitchin, there was an isolated hamlet near Ippollitts Brook called The Riddy and the furlong Riddy Shot bordered the brook. Other place names using this local term include Golden Riddy, Row Riddy Stream and the rather marvellous Duck Riddy.

Walking down Riddy Lane, I think of the Hitchin botanist, Joseph Edward Little, who wrote about the derivation of 'Riddy' in one of a series of articles on local place names in *The Hertfordshire Express* in 1927. Of all the naturalists I've researched, Joseph is the person I'd most like to have met. Born in Tonbridge in 1861, he moved to Hitchin in 1889 to take up the position of headmaster at the grammar school. He was a renowned field botanist, a specialist in willows, poplars and sedges, and he spent many years studying plants in and around Purwell Ninesprings, my local patch. Joseph began his nature journals in 1910 and continued writing into the 1920s, so I've been able to retrace some of his walks almost exactly one century on. I share his enthusiasm for the derivation of place names and the minutiae of paths, and I love to read his evocative descriptions, such as the reference to a broad-leaved osier (a hybrid willow) which he found on a track near Ninesprings 'about a third of the way down, just above where Mr Hailey's tram used to cross the ditch to the field of currant bushes'.

Joseph died at his home in Hitchin in January 1935, only a few minutes after revising his article 'On the migratory habit of some British Orchids'. I often stop to tell him the latest about our local patch as I pass his resting place in Hitchin Cemetery, where, come spring, the white flowers of meadow saxifrage speckle his grave – a sight which I'm sure would have pleased him.

On 31 July 1914, Joseph spotted yellow vetch growing in the wurzel field below Riddy Lane and, in one of my favourite extracts from his journals in 1910, he recorded some algae in a pond along the lane, likely at the place where he described a spring vanishing into a swallow hole. He queried:

Closterium? lunula: circulation observed in extremity of frond in transparent globular part free of chlorophyll.

His drawing of this desmid, or unicellular inhabitant of shallow, unpolluted freshwater, looks a little like a sausage with a lopsided, cheeky grin, but is in fact a rendering of two mirrored half-cells joined by a connecting section in which the cellular nucleus sits. I was particularly pleased to see that the website of the Dutch Desmid working group gave *Closterium lunula* the honour of being Desmid of the Month in October 2006. I doubt I'll meet this endearing alga as I wander down Riddy Lane, now surrounded by houses, no floodplain, marshy ground or ponds to be seen, but Joseph's entry, along with his hand-drawn maps and copious notes on the water-loving willows, sedges and rushes of Ninesprings, Ash Brook and Folly Alder Swamp, remind me of the watery nature of my area. Following in his soggy footsteps along the snickets, I feel a profound connection with the natural history of my local patch.

I sometimes wonder why my mind and feet lead me instinctively to the margins, why I have such an affinity with edgelands and snickets. Perhaps it's because I feel comfortable out of the limelight, somewhere where I can observe, unobserved.

Certainly, snickets can be inconspicuous, intimate places, but they're also subversive, rejecting the imposition of impermeable boundaries. I like the way they challenge our unconscious acceptance of facile dichotomies.

At school I sat on the academic fence. Science, maths and natural history were always threatening to infiltrate my literary studies like trespassers skulking outside the back door. When I enrolled on the secondary teaching course after my degree, my contemporaries chose arts subsidiaries alongside their English course. I took mathematics. While they planned French and drama lessons, I caught up with some of the topics the other maths students had covered during their undergraduate courses. I enjoyed the challenge. It was part of my attempt to see the world slant, to escape the pressure to pledge allegiance to one side or the other. Why choose arts or sciences when both fascinated me? Why ring-fence subjects rather than investigate the ways in which each discipline networked with its neighbour? I couldn't understand why the education system seemed so yoked to specialism, so incurious about the interconnectedness of things, being as I was an unabashed pluralist.

As part of my MA in the early 2000s, I had the opportunity to explore interdisciplinary studies in more depth. I investigated the influence of relativity and quantum theory on modernist literature, focusing on novelist Ford Madox Ford's First World War tetralogy, *Parade's End*. Ford seemed an ideal writer for this kind of study, as he questioned the credibility of science (his third wife said he didn't believe a word of it), yet he maintained close links with writers such as Wyndham Lewis, Joseph Conrad and Ezra Pound, all of whom explored contemporary scientific and philosophical ideas in their work. Despite Ford's alleged disdain for science, he experimented with all manner of stylistic and structural techniques related to changing perceptions of time, space and reality. With Ford's work in mind, I thought as I wrote my thesis, how could anyone dismiss the power of the zeitgeist – what he described as 'a veritable bacteriologist's soup for the culture of modern germs' – that wondrous and undeniable interconnectedness of life?

A few years later, after we had moved down south, I was invited to join the Cambridge University Science and Literature reading group. It was a revelation to meet other academics who were interested in connections between subjects. Among the texts up for discussion were *We*, a dystopian novel by Yevgeny Zamyatin set in a civilisation organised according to mathematical rules, and Edwin A. Abbott's *Flatland: A Romance in Many Dimensions*, a satirical novella set primarily in a two-dimensional world. Reading books that used geometrical landscapes and mathematical concepts to create symbolism and satire was utterly mind-bending. It rewrote my notions about the boundaries of the novel. Around the same time, I was asked to write my first piece of journalism – an article arguing the case for interdisciplinary studies in education. As I edged my way round the academic circle in both directions, I never imagined I would meet myself on the other side two decades later, writing about nature, landscape, gardens and literature. And that in those margins, I'd find integration and belonging.

On Pinehill Path, one of the back alleys into town, snicket life is on the move, engaging in marginal manoeuvres that challenge the suburban status quo. Austrian clematis coils over a wall and tumbles onto the path, freed from the rigours of trellis and twine. Its leaf stalks tangle with its wild cousin, old man's beard, which is on a reverse mission to infiltrate the cottage borders from the hedgerows. Both plants thrive in our calcareous soils; to them, scaling the wall is like scrambling through the subalpine vegetation or climbing high into the alder canopy. It matters little that this wall is a boundary denoting enclosure and possession or that the Austrian clematis is a favoured ornamental and wild *Clematis vitalba* a troublesome outsider. These climbers are merely travelling through the snickets, challenging the dichotomy we set up between culture and nature, revealing the absurd attitude of 'us and them': *Look up, they say, no matter how high you build, you can't tame us – we exist on both sides of your walls.*

Old man's beard certainly has no compunction about marking its territory in every part of the chalklands. I became familiar with this tenacious climber when I moved to Hertfordshire. Our first garden was laced with wiry coils disappearing up into the mature hazel tree, festooning the canopy with bearded achenes or single-seeded fruits that shed their softness over our heads as we tugged the lines down to free the branches above. In the alder carr (from the old Norse for 'marsh', referring to a boggy woodland) between houses and field edges, I saw the power of this airy climber en masse as its stems encircled slender alders, lignifying into vast networks of trunk and vine that I could only untwist in my mind through following the profligate trails to their extremities – roots in the chalk and silken seed heads lit up against the sky.

Following old man's beard soon became part of the daily routine. Equally at home twining through hedges as it is climbing trees, an individual plant can extend up to 30 metres. Stems can grow 2 metres a year, embracing everything in their paths. The more time I spent walking beside the entwined trails of old man's beard, the more my own adventitious roots extended, tentatively at first, then more firmly down into the chalky soil. Sixteenth-century writer and herbalist John Gerard coined another common name – 'traveller's joy' – in response to the plant's habit of 'decking and adorning waies and hedges, where people trauel', and Robert Frost's friend, the poet Edward Thomas, noted 'traveller's joy buds' in the hedges west of Hitchin on his meditative walk along the Icknield Way in 1911. His detailed descriptions of hedgerows epitomised his emphasis on journey rather than destination. In *The Icknield Way*, at the opening of chapter one 'On roads and footpaths', Thomas writes:

Much has been written of travel, far less of the road. Writers have treated the road as a passive means to an end, and honoured it most when it has been an obstacle; they leave the impression that a road is a connection between two points which only exists when the traveller is upon it.

Old man's beard, or traveller's joy, focuses the walker's attention on the pleasures of the journey through its very name and its habit of accompanying you along the way. Indeed, there's something companionable about the plant in every season: its chalky-white flowers, plump buds and feathery seed heads carry your eye along the verges, integrating disparate elements into a familiar whole. And wild clematis is just one of so many plants and animals that can be seen in the snickets. These days my walks are all about the more-than-human lives I meet along the way and the stories they tell.

Further up Pinehill Path, young elms have broken through a line of old fence panels and are busy creating thickets in an abandoned garden. In this unruly corner, corky elm saplings morph from planted field specimens to wild escapees to garden intruders in one single snicket-metre, suckering and blurring boundaries as they go. I've never known elm as a mature woodland tree, never seen its pinkish-red flowers or bunched samaras – its winged fruits. Had I lived here four centuries ago, elm would have been the predominant tree. A survey of land in the Manor of Hitchin in 1608 recorded 3,803 elms, 425 trees listed as either elm or ash, 155 ashes and 27 oaks. I can't begin to imagine what a landscape with this abundance of elms would look like. As it is, I've learned to identify its serrated leaves relatively recently on low-growing wayside specimens and often notice spindly suckers poking out of hedge bottoms.

What I wouldn't give to admire the Huntingdon elm that Joseph Edward Little described at Pinehill as 'a young tree in the field, with room to develop symmetrically' in the early 1920s. Suppose this sapling were now a century into its maturity, towering a majestic 30 metres above Pinehill Field, with post-football picnickers gathered under its canopy. Imagine walking beside the forgotten namesakes of Elmside, Elm Lodge and Elm Cottages, or looking down, as Joseph did from Royston Heath in North Hertfordshire, 'upon a line of Huntingdon elms in the direction of the station' in a year when 'the elms fruit[ed] so abundantly that for a time they ha[d] no energy left for the production of leaves'. Instead, throughout the UK, the extant elm names linked to houses, farms and estates are loosening their grip as our collective memories erode, while all along the hedgerows and snickets, elmlings lie low and sucker, spreading horizontally alongside old man's beard, keeping their crowns safely below the parapet.

At the other extreme, soaring above the train bridge just before the snicket folds between a line of hawthorn hedges and back fences, there's a thin slit of sky, a window offering passage into a brave new world. As the children grew older, they learned to identify the song thrush that called from the top of the ash trees; the blackcap with its seasonal territory on the south embankment and nest deep in the blackthorn scrub; the soft brush of foliage across the railings as the tallest ash emerged from beneath the bridge footings, reaching high above our heads. For years, this slender ash had been one of my daily companions, a quiet presence to nod to as I passed or lightly brush fingers to leaves in silent greeting. It was this ash which first displayed the telltale lesions and hanging shrivelled leaflets of ash dieback: a fungal disease that's killing ash trees across Europe. Perhaps the fungal spores had been carried to Hitchin in the slipstream of a passing train or on high winds. I knew it was only a matter of time once the disease was first recorded in the UK in 2012. I watched the train bridge ash closely for weeks, willing it to fight and send the fungus back down south via Thameslink or the London North Eastern Railway, but the foliage continued to wilt and eventually, following government guidance, I rang the notification line and reported the tree to the council.

Like snickets, ash trees are underappreciated, or at least were until their nemesis, ash dieback, arrived on our doorstep. Oliver Rackham lamented the tree's marginal status in *The Ash Tree*, explaining 'it has not the glamour of birch, the mystery of lime, the ruggedness of black poplar, the antiquity of yew, the magic of rowan, or the lore and legend of oak. It is a very recognisable tree that people are fond of in a quiet way, but not one that people are moved to write books about.' But now we're thinking about the importance of ash and facing a new reality without our commonest self-maintained tree (one still able to reproduce by seed in the wild).

As the helpline rang through, I had a strong compulsion to put the phone down and forget I'd seen those prematurely withered leaves. No one else knew. I'm not sure anyone else had even noticed the ash tree poking over the top of the bridge. But I'm an inveterate rule-follower, so I held the line until I was connected and then gave details of the tree's whereabouts. Feeling like I'd informed on a friend, the school run became a guilty affair, but the ash continued to brush my sleeve as I passed, still largely healthy despite the early warning signs. I convinced myself I'd made an error. No doubt the tree had already been inspected and found to be disease-free. Then, a week or two later, on one of my return journeys from the school run, emerging from thoughts of water bottles, cheerleading kit and pickup arrangements, I was suddenly aware of the absence of ash, like a gentle background noise you don't notice until it stops.

Now, all across the UK, ashes are falling silent, and with them the ecosystems that they can support throughout their long lives – around 200 years for a standard tree and 400 or more for coppiced specimens – the birds, bats, 111 species of insect and mite, the mosses, lichens and fungi and the herbaceous plants that thrive at the base of the ash canopy. It is devastating, this unremarkable hush, such an absence pooling, unnoticed, around the peripheries of our lives. I hear it now each time I cross the train bridge. It calls my attention to the narrow window the ash has left high above the tracks, through which there awaits a muted, thinner future.

Some snickets are more elusive, offering passage into the past only when you're ready to look. It can be years before that moment finally arrives. One day, walking down to Tesco Extra for emergency milk supplies, I crossed the road and climbed the bank to see what stage the blackthorn buds had reached. Perhaps one or two would be straining against the bud scales in an early intimation of spring. My mind was far away, still thinking about the three male bullfinches we'd seen the previous weekend eating blackthorn buds high in the hedges at Paxton Pits in Cambridgeshire, reflecting on the last time I'd seen bullfinches in the garden, the last time I'd rejoiced in their orange-meets-vermilion saturation and worried about the damage they might do to my blackcurrants. I realised it was more than ten years earlier and, even then, only a single bird. In Joseph Edward Little's notebook from 1908, he talks of yearly bellowings of bullfinches in his garden on my side of the town, but now, a century on, I might wait a decade between sightings.

Perhaps my fluid state of mind – a hundred years away and 2 metres up – unlocked the door: a narrow entrance marked with a wooden footpath sign which I must have passed hundreds, if not thousands of times on my daily commute to the train station. I could have sworn I'd never seen the sign or the gap in the hedge before. I walked past the entrance for a few days wondering which of us was the anachronism. But time and place remained stubbornly present and, eventually, I accepted that my inattention over all those years must have been behind this disconcerting revelation.

In my hazy mind-map, the houses beside the road bordered the railway embankment, but the presence of the overgrown snicket suggested otherwise. In fact, old maps reveal that this path joins up with the original road that led down by the railway when it opened in 1850. The snicket had perhaps offered passage to other walkers recently, judging by the sodden umbrella sleeve, balled-up wet wipes and cider cans discarded around the entrance, but I met no one, and the brambles that stretched between the ivied gateposts showed no signs of having been recently parted. Just inside the briar doorway, a single crocus stretched in purple-and-orange optimism towards the sky before its inevitable slump. Further along, beneath the privet fringes, small clusters of crocuses had reached the melancholic stage all too quickly, laying down their blown, flaccid heads down on the ivy, revealing naked white stems. Each slushy petal, still violet-smeared and flecked with orange stamens, was echoed on the embankment on the far side of the snicket by the bags of rubbish that had been tipped over the fence, their garish Dairy Milk and Fanta shades adding to the visual miscellany – three recycling boxes, a once-white interior door, the shed skin of a Spiderman balloon, a couple of tyres, a recumbent ironing board.

Ivy was marking time across the embankment, sifting the cast-offs into categories: recent (still resting on top of the vegetation), long-term (bound tightly by ivy tendrils) and bygone (practically submerged by vine-vigour). Like old man's beard, ivy's homogenising tendency was inciting collusion at the snicket edge. Where volunteer cotoneaster met cow parsley, lavender flirted with red dead-nettle, an incongruous Christmas tree sheltered Jack-by-the-Hedge, and aubretia rambled up the banks through wild marjoram and red valerian. Whether rising from the sea of lobed ivy leaves on the juvenile growth or cloaked in the older leathery foliage that climbed tree and fence post, wild and cultivated were bound together with the same commonplace identity.

I love the way climbers cross axes, scaling the vertical, bridging gaps, emerging as horizontal ground cover. And they are not tenacious simply in three dimensions, they have temporal roots too. Old man's beard and ivy are indigenous plants, deeply anchored in local time, but along the railway banks there's a newer climber on the ascent. Broad-leaved everlasting pea threads through the undergrowth unnoticed until June coaxes out lipstick-pink blooms that overwhelm the eye but underwhelm the nose. Pull a flower through the railings and the sensory effect is as futile as if I had sniffed the dog-eared remains of the plastic bunch of flowers cable-tied to the railings on the snicket by the train bridge, presumably with its own sad history. Unlike its closely related wildflower cousin (the narrow-leaved everlasting pea), the broad-leaved everlasting pea is a garden escape that's been grown in the UK as an ornamental for centuries. Its ability to climb meant it soon escaped over the garden wall and became established in the wider landscape, particularly on railway embankments in the south of England. First recorded in the wild in Hertfordshire in 1874, by 1912 it was growing near Benslow Bridge, having in all likelihood escaped from Alfred Ransom's garden, which extended right up to the edge of the cutting. It has persisted on the embankment for over a century, jostling with old man's beard and ivy, all potential candidates for long-term, if not everlasting, survival.

Even at my contemplative pace (physically walking the path, mentally scrambling along the railway embankment with the climbers), I soon reached the end of the secret passage that had revealed itself to me a few days earlier. Stepping over brambles, I emerged past a row of 15 bins, a new Astroturf lawn and a paved stub of a front garden decorated with a scattering of ash-grey aggregate. Goldfinches burbled at the top of the conifer hedge. When I looked back, the snicket had dissolved into ivy.

The sudden appearance of the snicket along the railway embankment taught me that we don't notice what we don't expect to see. But I'm also learning it's not only physical doors into the past that remain hidden until you are ready to find them. Now, with both children settled at school and my collection of tales about the local landscape nearing completion, I'm as prepared as I'll ever be to make my way back to the forgotten years of my early childhood. I know by now that the relationship between the human and more-than-human world is a vital part of my story – that any way forward involves seeing myself – ourselves – as a part of nature rather than apart from it. Writing about the natural world as a way to escape my own life no longer seems a responsible choice. The only way forward is to look for the lost child. So, with the help of my counsellor, I search for an entrance into my own past. I find the door open, waiting for me, as if it had always been so.

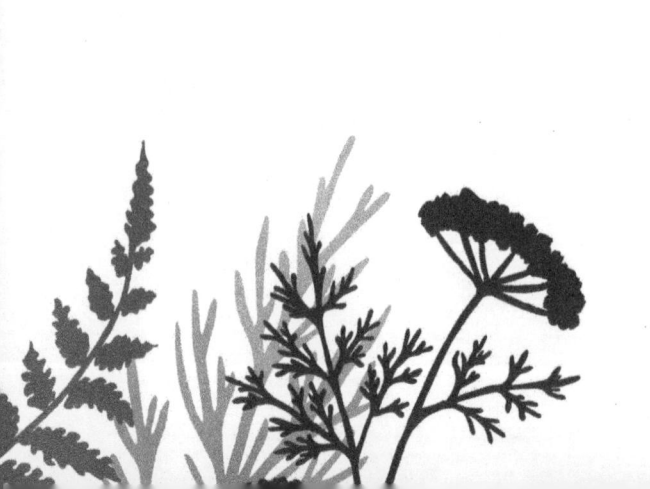

The Nightingale's Tale

To enter the world of memory is to take on the labyrinth. Time bends. Dimensions shift. The way is treacherous, the air thick with menace. I am seeking the lost child, that part of myself I wished away all those years ago. I know the truth is in here somewhere, but the longer I look, the more disoriented I become. And all the while – around the next corner? at the top of the steps? – the Goblin King is waiting. His is the mocking voice in my head that warns me these memories are not mine for the taking. "This journey into the unknown," he taunts, "is nothing but self-indulgent fantasy."

I am appalled when I actually listen to these words for the first time. When I see how vehemently they deny my reality and suppress negative emotions from the past.

"You'll be judged and despised for telling stories to gain sympathy," he warns me, harking back to the way I saw myself as a child – as a contemptible attention-seeker – a belief closely connected to other people's attitudes towards Mum and her illness. I realise I stopped judging her in that way many years ago but forgot to extend the same courtesy to myself. It explains why I find writing about my own life so difficult.

So when I venture forth, I come forearmed with moments from the past extracted from boxes of letters, journals and diaries, from medical records, photo albums and recorded conversations, the tapes we made for my grandma when I was a child and, more recently, reminiscences over drinks with my brother, childhood visits relived with my cousin, a summer's afternoon perusing old slides with my parents beside the River Lee. I gather my research and select my weapons. And then, with little to guide me but old facts and borrowed memories, I set out to find myself.

My journey into the labyrinth takes me back to the 1950s. The way ahead is straightforward, signposted with notes taken during a recent conversation with my parents. I tell my mother's story first, writing about the child rebuked for laziness; the student struggling with depression and illness; the mother gaslit by those who should have helped her, unable to feel any love for her baby daughter, barely able to crawl across the floor to get her a banana. I prefer not to think about the baby.

Progress is swift, though I am not sure I like where the narrative path is leading. But I have come too far to go back now, and besides, writing has become a compulsion. I find a way into my own past through familiar memories – good ones – of reading and playing, helping Dad in the garden, pantomimes and singing. There are no bad memories because my childhood was a happy one. At least that is what I believe, until suddenly I enter uncharted territory. Within a few paragraphs I have lost myself in shame, illness and withdrawal. I am astonished by the intensity of feeling that reveals itself on the page. Fear, sadness, confusion, self-loathing – old emotions forgotten for so long that it's hard to believe they were ever real, though they feel so visceral when I write. The facts about the severity of my mother's postnatal depression and chronic illness, most of which I discovered only once I started asking questions for the book, have taken months to sink in. Now I'm beginning to wonder about the effect of her illness on my childhood development. Feeling underhand, I do some research and learn that children who have not had their emotional needs met in early childhood are more vulnerable to dissociating as a survival mechanism. When I add up my history of anxiety, dissociation and the sense that I am profoundly flawed, the narrative seems to be leading to uncharitable conclusions. I start to feel horribly guilty. My writing seems a betrayal of loving parents who have always done their best for me. Who am I to think any difficulties I faced deserved attention or support? Everyone has tough experiences to deal with. For God's sake woman, pull yourself together and stop making such a fuss.

He is almost irresistible, the Goblin King in my head, presenting his insidious arguments with such conviction. He offers me anonymity and safety. All I need do is promise to abandon my journey. Turn back and forget. But I have had enough of ignorance and silence. I want to find a way to tell my story. With the support of my counsellor, I fight back. I challenge his injunctions and press forward regardless of the cost. I decide it is time to acknowledge the negative emotions in my childhood and see where they take me. Once I've allowed myself this freedom, it feels like committing my authentic self to the page for the very first time. This sense of having found my voice carries me into the next chapter and beyond, though I often waver and consider retreat when the incessant critic castigates me for reliving and sharing difficult experiences. Despite these delays, I plough on. I feel I am getting closer to an understanding of why, as an adult, I dissociate when experiencing anxiety and severe fatigue. I know now that the lost child holds the key.

By the end of chapter four, encouraged by my progress and ready for the next section, I come up against an uncomfortable truth. Until now I have been writing for myself, but if I want to publish, I must share my story with my mother. I must address difficult issues we have never talked about, because it is her story too. But I am desperately afraid my motives are selfish ones. What if finding my voice and improving my mental health comes at the expense of hers? What if I damage family relationships with my questions? Mum's emotional needs have always been greater than mine and that's all there is to it. Every time I think about sending her the chapters, all the work I've done with my counsellor unravels. I'm petrified she'll tell me it didn't happen that way. That my feelings of sadness, fear and shame are mere delusions. I put down my pen. The Goblin King is right. The only way forward is to turn back and forget.

As always when life becomes too difficult, I look to the natural world for inspiration. I'm in luck. It's early spring, so there's plenty happening outside to keep me busy. I watch a kingfisher plunge-diving for stickleback in the reedbed pond and spend a quiet afternoon top-dressing the pots in the garden with compost. Over the fields, skylarks sing and a smattering of lapwings exult in daredevil display flights. Unlike me, the natural world is making progress, seemingly more alive every day.

I walk outside as much as my energy levels allow and return to researching local natural history, enjoying the academic detachment it offers. One day, while browsing the British Newspaper Archives, I come across an article in the *Cardiff Evening Express* from 1898 entitled 'Praying for the Crops'. It wasn't unusual at this time for regional papers to cover stories from beyond their bounds, and the article describes the revival of the Rogation Day tradition in Hitchin, where clergy, choristers and congregation would make their way out to local fields and homesteads (in this case, those of nearby Walsworth and Purwell) to bless the crops with prayers and hymns. I read the account of the procession and the corn 'strong in the blade and of a very good colour' with interest, but it's the opening of the piece that catches my eye. Hitchin is described as 'an old-fashioned market town, some thirty miles from London, a district famous for its lavender and for its nightingales.' I know about the lavender, but not the nightingales. My curiosity is piqued.

I've never seen a nightingale in Hertfordshire. In fact, I'd only ever encountered the legendary songster in poetry and music before I moved down south. At university, I studied Keats's 'Ode To A Nightingale' and sang of love inspired by the nightingale's song: *'Liebe mich, geliebtes Herz / Küsse mich im Dunkeln!'* ('Love me, dear heart / Kiss me in the dark!') in Brahms's *Liebeslieder Walzer*. If I thought of nightingales back then, it was as aesthetic muses or romantic metaphors, not as birds of feather, blood and bone, of thickset hedge and scrubby woodland.

When we moved to Hitchin in January 2003, we rented a two-bed terrace just off Nightingale Road – a convenient location close to the train station. The Nightingale pub across the road had seen better days. Our walk into town passed Nightingale Cottages, two of the oldest properties in the north-east quarter of the town. Opening our bedroom sash window on summer evenings, we could hear birds warbling, whistling and trilling, flaunting their mimicry skills. Not nightingales, of course, but the day's soundbites replayed by the rooftop starlings. One specialised in mobile phone ringtones. It caught us out more than once and I missed its musical jingles when we moved.

In mid-April of that year, I saw my first nightingale on a family walk around Paxton Pits Nature Reserve in Cambridgeshire. Even though the reserve had 28 singing males, I felt lucky to see and hear this denizen of the understorey. It was also my granny's first encounter with a nightingale, a bird she had wanted to hear all her life. She finally achieved her wish two days after her eightieth birthday. A couple of weeks later, I set my alarm for 3.15 a.m. and joined a dawn chorus walk at Sandy, where I heard my second nightingale of the season. At Minsmere, at the end of May, I upped my tally to three.

In contrast to the nature reserves of Cambridgeshire, Bedfordshire and Suffolk, the landscape around my first rented house in Hitchin felt urban and uninspiring. Though I spent a couple of years surrounded by titular nightingales, it never occurred to me to wonder about the origins of the local road, pub and cottage names. And even if it had, there'd have been little information to go on. No one seems certain how Nightingale Road got its name. According to *Two Minutes to the Station*, a local history study of the area, the origins of the road are 'lost in the mists of time'. But now, with the Cardiff newspaper article in mind, I'm curious to know if there's more to the old place names than I thought. I start to search for Hitchin's nightingales in earnest, an ornithological pilgrimage that provides a welcome distraction from my personal narrative with all its detours, delays and dead ends.

The earliest record I can find is from 16 April 1811. On this spring day in Hitchin, over two centuries ago, Joseph Ransom, a 26-year-old Quaker, noted in his *Naturalist's Notebook*: 'Wrynecks, Redstarts, Nightingales & Blackcaps have all arrived within these few days.' Seventy-seven years later, the first Hitchin nightingale of the season was recorded in the journal of the Hertfordshire Natural History Society on 18 April by Alfred Ransom, Joseph's nephew. Alfred lived in Benslow House, on the opposite side of Benslow Lane to his younger brother, William. Nightingales sang in Alfred's pleasure grounds, perhaps in the trees his father had planted on the hill a generation earlier. If I'd been labouring in Purwell Field 150 years ago, in the spot where my house now stands, their strident song would have carried to me across the newly built railway line.

The Natural History Society journal recorded the dates of natural phenomena every year in the interests of science. 'Who does not listen for the first note of the nightingale?' members were asked in 1876. 'Who does not look out for the first swallow? Who cannot help saying, once a year at least, "There's the cuckoo!"' Even the county's youth were seen as valuable contributors. Children should be trained, members were advised, 'to observe the blossoming of wildflowers, and to look out for the arrival of birds, etc., which observations might be recorded by their parents and sent to the Society.'

Reading through the journals from the late nineteenth century to the present day is like pressing fast forward on a disaster movie. In 1877, Hertfordshire corn miller and respected ornithologist John Littleboy read his paper 'The Birds of Our District' to the society. Littleboy noted that the nightingale 'generally reaches this district between the 10th and 21st of April' and recounted the story of a relative who had induced three nightingales to come for food whenever she called them. In 1884, he reported that the birds were 'less abundant' and, by 1889, nightingales were becoming scarcer in the county every year, perhaps partly because:

> no bird is more easily caught by that pernicious race the birdcatchers than the nightingale, and, though sold at a high price, on none is their cruelty more gratuitously exercised.

Around the turn of the century, Hertfordshire's nightingales were 'either very scarce or very silent' and, in 1913, the county bird recorder William Bickerton noted sadly that:

> References to the Queen of British songsters (though it is the male bird that sings, and not his queen) become less and less frequent in the reports that reach me as the years go by, so I am afraid there is no doubt that the bird is getting scarcer in Hertfordshire. This is certainly true for the Watford district, for I do not now hear a tenth of the numbers of nightingales in song as I did some eight or ten years ago. Coppices and spinneys which always contained their annual pair are

now tenantless of nightingales, though the immediate surroundings of such former haunts are in no way changed. It is difficult to account for their gradual disappearance.

The fading of the nightingale's song seems to me an ironic reflection of the Greek myth of Procne, Queen of Thrace, and her sister, Philomela. Procne is married to King Tereus, who rapes Philomela and cuts out her tongue to ensure her silence. Philomela weaves her tale into a tapestry and the sisters enact revenge by killing Tereus's son. As the king chases the women, they transform into birds – in Ovid's version of the tale, Procne into a swallow and her sister, a nightingale. Thus, Philomela escapes and acquires a new voice with which to recount her sad history. Perhaps her lament, where it could still be heard in Hertfordshire, took on a new resonance for listeners at the beginning of the twentieth century if they recalled the abundance of past decades.

A general population decrease was noted across West Hertfordshire in the 1930s, and nightingales were said to have decreased in many localities by 1959. Breeding was recorded through the 1960s and 70s, though the species was listed as 'status decreasing'. By the time of the BTO survey in 1980, only 21 singing males were recorded in the county. These figures showed a reduction of almost 90 per cent within a decade. Their precipitous decline was linked to the disappearance of almost all woodland under coppice management and the loss of damp scrub. The last breeding record in the county was in 1994. The latest Hertfordshire State of Nature report continues the sorry story. Between 1970 and 2020, my adopted county witnessed the extinction of 76 animal and plant species – including the nightingale. That's more than three species every two years. The first year in which not a single nightingale was heard or recorded anywhere in Hertfordshire was 2003. By 2005, the idea of finding them nesting in the county was described as 'wishful thinking'.

Once widespread across Hertfordshire, and very abundant in some areas, this iconic bird is now extinct as a breeding species in the county. My kids could spend every hour of every spring exploring the osier scrub along the River Purwell, where nightingales used to sing, and never hear a note. We love to play among the bluebells in Hitch Wood, but we are not serenaded by wood warblers trilling in the oaks as we might have been a century ago. We wander down Riddy Lane, but see no mice, bumblebees or linnets impaled on thorns in the larders of breeding red-backed shrikes. Shopping in town along Hermitage Road, once part of Frederic Seebohm's land, we will not spot a hawfinch nest like the one ornithologist Henry Seebohm wrote about seeing in his brother's garden in *A History of British Birds* in 1884. As we walk along Gypsy Lane beside the reedbeds, I tell the children that 40 years ago tree sparrows would have been chittering in the elm trees that also died decades ago. We have silenced so many species, yet we barely notice their absence. The concept of abundance does not haunt us in the way it should. I cannot help wondering what our children have done to deserve this ghostly legacy.

My parents are sifting through the contents of their loft now they've moved from Cheshire to Bedfordshire to be nearer their children and grandchildren. Even though I've stopped writing, Mum keeps sending me snippets of information gleaned from old photographs and documents. She finds the letters she and Dad wrote to each other when they were going out, and a picture of me aged six or so, dressed in green velour shorts and white socks, holding a young lamb tightly against my bare tummy while an unknown hand feeds it from a bottle. I'm smiling, minus one front tooth. She emails me old names she's learned for siskins: 'black-headed thistle finch' and 'golden wren'. I'm grateful for her help; I just wish I was writing the story she thinks I am. Perhaps then I'd feel able to share my chapters with her.

I'm struck, on rereading her messages, by the realisation that my love of the natural world comes from both my parents, not just my father. When I think back to childhood, every memory concerning the garden or wildlife centres around me and Dad. We chat in the veg patch, go orienteering in the woods, watch birds in the trees. But now I'm not so sure my mum was absent all the time. I think I've erased her from some of these memories. I certainly know that she shared her love of music with me and encouraged my eclectic approach to the arts. When I sang onstage in the pantomimes, Mum was there playing the piano or sitting in the audience. She went to my parents' evenings and watched *Neighbours* with me when I came home from school. I'm not sure why I've accepted her absence from almost all of my happy memories without question. Perhaps repressed anger ripped out the good times while I looked the other way – old anger I couldn't process, because, even as a young child, it felt unfair to blame someone for something that was not their fault. But neither was it mine. And suppressing the anger suppressed the good memories too.

Accessing some of these old emotions doesn't mend the rips or fill the gaps, but it does enable me to let go. Though I can't see her face when I look back across the years, I know she was there. There were, without doubt, long periods of absence and illness, a worrying unpredictability to life that never went away. Days and weeks when she couldn't cope with seeing us, when everything I said to try and help seemed to make things worse. But there was also love and laughter and kindness, and I can feel my anger turning to regret. Any remaining negative emotions are directed towards the medical system that routinely gaslit my mother and failed to offer the support she needed in those early months of postnatal depression, after which I suspect the damage to our mother–daughter bond had already been done.

I feel extremely lucky that we have a good adult relationship. My mother has changed a great deal since I was a child, though sadly she still lives with ME/CFS. And I am changing too. If she were well right now, I might consider sending her the chapters. But he's tenacious, the Goblin King. As soon as the way forward seems clear, he changes the rules. Mum's physical health has deteriorated over the last few months, and she's spent much of her time in bed. This long spell of illness has inevitably taken its toll on her ability to cope. The last thing I want is to cause more suffering. It's a risk I'm not willing to take. That's when I realise my journey through the labyrinth has reached its final dead end.

The nightingale's tale continues to be a compelling distraction. I've learned how the species became extinct in Hertfordshire but still have no proof of their erstwhile fame in Hitchin. I carry on researching, not expecting to find much. The next reference comes from a most unexpected source. In the spring of 1882, the American literary naturalist John Burroughs (who would go on to become good friends with John Muir and Theodore Roosevelt) visited the UK. After spending the latter half of May in Scotland, he travelled through northern England and down to the South. In his essay 'A Hunt for the Nightingale' published a couple of years later, he explains that hearing the song of the nightingale is one of the chief pleasures he has promised himself on the trip. Unfortunately, by the time he reaches the bushy fields and overgrown hedgerows around Haslemere, in the south-west corner of Surrey, it is already 17 June. A local farmer tells him he is too late, but Burroughs refuses to be disheartened.

In the gloaming, he hovers around copses and hedgerows 'like one meditating a dark deed'. He thrills to the *Jr-r-r-r-r* or *Chr-r-r-r-r* of the nightjar and enjoys the solitary nocturne of the sedge warbler, whose whimsical performance continues until after midnight. The following afternoon, he embarks upon a pilgrimage through the dusky groves, copses and thickets of Surrey and Hampshire in pursuit of the nightingale's song. Along the way, he takes a walk with a taxidermist's errand boy who assures him the swallow that skims along the road in front of them is a nightingale, and hears the 'chiding, guttural note' of what he thinks is his quarry in bushes near a house but is forced to retreat lest the woman at the window thinks he has designs upon her home. He meets country folk who recount stories of the nightingales they have heard in recent hours; shivers under a pine tree with only midges for company in a spot where a nightingale sings every night, but hears only a smattering of warm-up notes;

requests a bed at a series of inns with little success; hears a single nightingale note beside the River Wey and then no more; and journeys to Selborne having convinced himself that Gilbert White's haunts will provide the one sound he most longs to hear. After two rainy, nightingale-less days loitering along 'wet lanes and dells and dripping hangers, wooing both [his] bird and the spirit of the gentle parson, but apparently without getting very near to either,' he walks to Alton and catches the train to London.

Not wanting to admit defeat, the next day he takes the train towards Cambridge and gets off at a 'large picturesque old town' where he thinks himself 'in just the right place at last.' Burroughs has chosen Hitchin for his final attempt to track down his elusive quarry. He walks to a road 'between the station and the town proper called Nightingale Lane, famous for its songsters' and asks at a 'thrifty-looking inn on the corner' (where he is once again refused bed and food) where he might hear nightingales. The innkeeper tells Burroughs he often sits with his friends listening to their music through his open windows. They sing morning and night in the trees opposite the inn, and the last time he heard them was only the previous evening. Burroughs, hoping for a melodic dénouement and with nowhere to sleep, spends the night wandering the streets like a patrolman listening out for snatches of song. By morning, he has caught nothing but neuralgic pains in his shoulder. However, he concludes:

It matters little, after all; I have seen the country and had some object for a walk, and that is sufficient.

So ends Burroughs's hunt for the nightingale, but not mine. By this point, I am more than intrigued. If the American naturalist journeyed to Hitchin in his final attempt to see nightingales, it would seem their fame had indeed spread far and wide. But what had become of Nightingale Lane and the thrifty-looking inn?

I found the first answer in a letter sent to the *Hertfordshire Mercury and Reformer* in November 1888, complaining that old and appropriate street names around Hitchin were being supplanted by new names of a more 'high-sounding character'. The writer recommended changing these back again, in particular the 'glaring instance' of 'Nightingale-lane', which she explained:

> got that name, I believe, because for many years a nightingale has sung regularly in the spring season in one part of the hedge.

Nightingales tend to be faithful to their breeding sites, so this could, for a few years at least, have been the same bird. The majority of male youngsters return to their natal areas to nest, so the territory was likely occupied for the period she mentions, and perhaps far longer, by birds that had hatched in or around the lane.

According to *The Street Names of Hitchin,* Nightingale Lane had also been known as Green Lane or Love Lane, suggesting it was a secluded, rural spot before the area was developed in the wake of the railway. Was it infamous for lovers' trysts, or was it the song of the nightingale, which for many centuries had been associated with romantic love and sexual liaisons, that gave the lane its amorous reputation? We will almost certainly never know. Nevertheless, these names offer an insight into the natural and social history of the area. Once the lane was renamed Verulam Road in 1883, a year after Burroughs's visit, the memory of the old and appropriate names and their meanings would have gradually faded away.

The question of what happened to the thrifty-looking inn takes me back to my early days in Hitchin. Its location on the corner of what used to be Nightingale Lane suggests Burroughs visited the Radcliffe Arms, my local pub when I lived in the area. Here, I chatted in the bar with friends after choir practice and, in later years, met up with a group of local parents, one of whom managed the pub, to share the highs and lows of living with little ones while our toddlers caused havoc around customers' feet.

An exploration of the history of the Radcliffe Arms seems to confirm my suspicions. Victorian newspaper reports refer to a Nightingale Inn situated on the corner of Nightingale Lane from at least 1855 (when the innkeeper gave evidence at a garrotting robbery) until 1865, when it became the Radcliffe Arms. Burroughs had unwittingly called at the Nightingale Inn 17 years after it was renamed, and spoken to Thomas Spencer, the innkeeper. It seems Burroughs's instinct for nightingale territory was spot on, even if his luck was not.

I find a couple of other references to Hitchin's famous nightingales too, such as an 1884 article in *Hardwicke's Science Gossip*, a popular science magazine, which refers to the fact that 'Hitchin claims to be a favourite spot for the nightingale, and can even boast of a "nightingale road,"' and a reference by local naturalist and prolific writer William Percival Westell in 1918 to hearing a chiffchaff from Hermitage Road in the area that still had breeding hawfinches. He notes:

if, as I am informed by a reliable authority, Hitchin has to mourn the loss of some of its famous Nightingales, compensation is forthcoming in the presence of the Chiff-Chaff and Hawfinch, to say nothing of the Rooks and Jackdaws, which are such a feature of the bird-life of the old market town.

I am astonished that we lived for two and a half years in an area so famous in the 1880s for its nightingales that it enticed the most popular American nature writer of the time to visit, yet never knew. An internet search for 'Hitchin famous for' lists the birthplace of the Queen Mother, the lavender fields, historic buildings, music festivals and the medieval wool trade. But where architecture, farming, agriculture, music and royalty all feature as notable examples of civic pride, natural history, naturalists and nightingales are nowhere to be found. The memories we choose to celebrate and remember, and those we allow to fade away, reveal much about what we value as a society. The tale of Hitchin's nightingales is simply one example of the disappearance of a species and the subsequent erosion of its memory. We did not just oust them – we forgot they ever existed.

My ornithological pilgrimage is at an end. It leaves me with a new ache for what we've destroyed and forgotten, and a keen desire to tell the nightingale's tale, both locally and in my book, as an example of how easily precious knowledge can pass out of living memory. It occurs to me that my pilgrimage through old records to uncover the history of Hitchin's wildlife is not so dissimilar to my personal quest into my childhood after all. In both cases, I'm looking for forgotten information that will help explain the present and perhaps lead to better choices in the future. As I consider the nightingale's tale and its relevance to my own personal history, I realise how vital it is to remember.

This thought brings me back to the first four chapters of my book. I've spent so much time lost in labyrinthine anxiety and guilt. It needs to stop. There has to be a way to beat the voice that denies my reality. My counsellor and friends are right. I must have more faith in the integrity of my emotions. At the end of March, I finally muster up my courage and confront the Goblin King. I tell him he has no power over me. Then I email my mother.

I explain that the book I'm writing is not the one I set out to write. She knows that having experimented with sections on landscape and nature for a few years, I finally recognised the need to put myself in the narrative. But now I confess that when I began to explore my relationship with chronic illness and anxiety, I felt like my life had fallen apart. I tell her I've been having counselling for the past seven months and that writing and counselling are helping me address physical and mental health issues that I've spent decades trying to ignore. I explain that I'm learning to own negative emotions as well as positive ones, that my writing feels transformative, as if releasing me from years of fear, sadness and shame. I tell her how worried I've been about the way my book might affect her and Dad, that some of the stuff I've had to deal with has been tough because we – particularly Mum, but the rest of the family too – were left in a cruel and impossible situation as a result of the way society and the medical profession treated illnesses it didn't acknowledge or understand. Then I ask if she would mind reading the first four chapters of my book.

When her reply arrives in my inbox later in the day, I am crying and shaking so violently that I cannot read the words. I have repressed my feelings for so long – those I have been able to access – believing I was protecting myself, or both of us, working on patterns of behaviour laid down in childhood, that giving voice to my emotions feels unbelievably transgressive. When I finally calm down enough to focus on the screen, I realise I have misjudged the situation. Mum's response is kind, supportive and... surprising. She refers, for the first time, to the way she feels she neglected me as a baby and child, more emotionally than physically, and to her sadness at what happened and its subsequent effect on our relationship.

Over the next few days, Mum reads the chapters and tells me she completely validates all I have written. She writes about her illness and the love she was unable to express in the first 15 months of my life. She sends me all the hugs she was never able to give me and those she gave later that I was not able to receive. She explains how, when I was 15 months old, I looked at her and said "Mummy" and she felt the first sudden explosion of love for me. She tells me how well she thinks I've done to have become such a balanced person despite all the difficulties thrown at me as a child.

Her words are a gift. Though writing the chapters has been painful, it is such a relief to discover the reason for those missing seven years, the dissociation, the unaccountable feelings of sadness and fear, my inability to remember her kindness, the pervasive sense that something was badly wrong with me. Looking back over my concerns about showing her my writing, I see the fears of my seven-year-old self. The child who was afraid she would make her mother sad or angry, and that her mother's illness would be her fault.

But rather than being upset, Mum says she is simply glad it has helped me to write it. Her words make me realise I no longer need to repress difficult emotions to protect myself or anyone else. The way forward now is to talk honestly about how I feel. Writing and counselling have helped me fight the Goblin King. I have navigated the labyrinth and found the frightened child, but she is not me anymore. She is just a memory. I draw her onto my lap and comfort her as I would my own daughter. "Everything will be okay," I say. Then I kiss her on the head and leave her in the past.

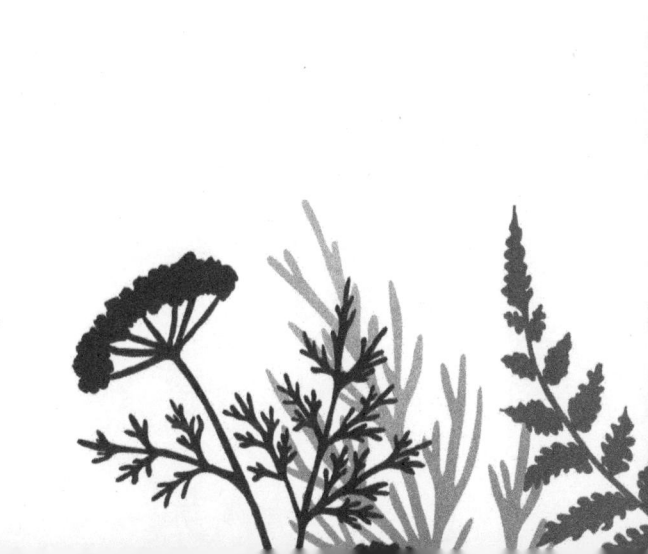

After weeks of January rain, water seeps back out of the saturated land. I'm reminded of a recurring dream where my garden rests on a fragile crust above an infinite cavern. Sinkholes open without warning, threatening to pitch the whole garden – lawn, borders, shed and all – down to goodness-knows-where. Just as I think the rifts are healing, my children run out to play, heeding my advice to get some fresh air, and away they tumble. I follow them in my mind's eye, falling through eternity: a descent that passes beyond the threshold of imagination. I wake with sickness coating my heart. In daylight, the garden looks calm and whole. But the landscape is mercurial and I do not trust my step.

Inundation

Mid-July, on the day of my wedding anniversary, my first country diary column comes out in *The Guardian*. It is my passport to a wilder life. In the couple of years since the children have both been at school, I've been straying from the snickets, making for the alder carr, water meadows and chalk streams whenever I can, learning where the sedge warbler sings and the redwings forage, making friends with the trees, hunting for the first marsh orchids of the season. And wherever I go, my guilty conscience follows. I feel like a shirker, dreaming in the meadows while other mums clean the house, visit the gym or return to work. While they stand around chatting at school pickup, looking smart in Lycra or work clothes, I pitch up late in my wellies, picking twigs and ladybirds out of my hair. Rather than returning to work, I've invented some Bohemian nonsense about being a writer.

I'm sure my upbringing influences my feeling that I ought to find a sensible job. I come from generations of no-nonsense working-class women on my mum's maternal side, grafters who disapproved of idleness but also, ironically, struggled with energy-limiting conditions. Our family's work ethic was no doubt linked to poverty, but I wonder if society's condemnation of female lethargy, depression and so-called hysteria also played a part. I recall very little about my nana (my great-grandmother) except she hummed tunelessly to music only she could hear, as if she already half-belonged to another world. She died, aged 91, when I was nine. Nana had bipolar disorder. She struggled with severe fatigue and was thought to be lazy by those around her. In the early 1960s, she was treated with electroconvulsive therapy. Her sister died of pernicious anaemia, an autoimmune disorder that causes, among other symptoms, extreme fatigue and weight loss. I wonder if attitudes towards her and her sister's conditions influenced family beliefs about hard work. My childhood experience of responses to Mum's 'idleness' certainly made me critical of my own need for rest, solitude and creative space. It might not stop me stealing time out in the wetlands once both kids are at school, but it exacerbates my guilt.

When I begin to write professionally about the natural world, I feel as if my interests and pleasures have been ratified. Now, when I potter and think and write, I can claim to be working. When I lose track of time watching banded demoiselles by the ford or return home too late to cook dinner after a parcel of linnets waylay me in the horse paddock, I cut myself some slack. It is a liberating feeling, except in its antithesis. Why did I not allow myself this personal and creative freedom before? Why did I dismiss wandering and dreaming as mere child's play, an unseemly pursuit for a busy mum with a million socks to pair? I wish I could have left those repressive attitudes in the past.

The more time I spend in the wetlands, the more I come to love and rely on them, especially the chalk stream and reedbeds that I dismissed as not wild enough when I moved here, which says more about my lack of vision than the landscape's lack of wildness. I think I love my patch most in the darker months when common snipe return to the water meadows. When the rains come and the land disappears underwater. When reedbed ponds overflow and merge, and intermittent springs bubble up in the boggy fields and alder carr. When I feel uprisings beneath me as the chalkland dreams of returning to sea.

One night, the holloway skirting the meadows reverts to river. I wade in, feeling the pressure of water against my wellies. In the darkness beside the ditch, I could be miles from the shore. The best way to travel, I decide as I test the riverbed for footholds, would be by coracle. Launched into the spring-fed flow, drifting downstream fishing for fallen moonbeams in the floodwater.

By the light of day, it appears the land *is* on the move. The reedbeds are steeped in a milky viridian green. I wonder how much of the turbidity is caused by chalky topsoil swilling off the fields into the overflowing ditches. All around my feet, slivers of sky are brought down to earth. Rain upends reality and emulsifies time. I think of the area's former name: Rushmead. Of labourers scything water meadows when the floodplain extended across the valley. I know the rhythmical swing of the scythe, the prickle on the back of the neck as cut vegetation is shouldered away. I've cleared reeds and scythed wet meadows, working alongside brush cutters, which speed up the process. No such help was available for Purwell reed cutters in the past though. All the meadows and reedbeds would have been cut by hand, the rushes and reeds sold in Hitchin for basketry, mats and thatching.

During cold winters, a century or more ago, the frozen water meadows would have lured out the town's skaters. As a child I learned about river skating from the scene in *Tom's Midnight*

Garden where Tom and Hatty ice-skate all the way from Castleford (Cambridge) to Ely, in the glacial winter of 1895. I didn't realise, though, that fen skating was a popular winter pursuit in East Anglia during the nineteenth century, and presumably in some of the outlying fens in Hertfordshire too, when the floodplains froze over. Imagine the glissando of skates on ice! Wind whipping hair and chafing cheeks. The ecstasy of flying over solid ground that only days ago mired you in sludge.

But such exhilaration in the wetlands was not without its dangers. While thawing ice on the water meadows might at worst give you a chilling dip, mistaking the state of rivers and lakes could have fatal consequences. In February 1895, around the time that Tom and Hatty were supposedly skating to Ely, the great frost claimed the life of many revellers, including Frederick Collens, an 18-year-old who drowned when he plunged through the ice while skating on Rostherne Mere in Cheshire.

Every watery story I hear and every walk I take, every volunteer session scything, ditch-clearing or hedge-laying, binds me closer to the wetlands:

Right here, see the vigorous regrowth on this hazel I coppiced four years ago.

Over there I was stopped in my tracks by the blaze of a red underwing moth resting on the debarked trunk of that dead black poplar.

Here's the spot where the children and I travelled by hand lens into a lichenous world of adventure, and where some enterprising youngsters built the homeliest of dens.

Nod when you reach the boardwalk, a courtesy to the alderman of the woods. See there, with a woodpecker h-O-le of a mouth and that twiglet wave?

Here in the wet meadow, a male whitethroat sang proudly from the bramble patch all spring.

A blackcap built one of his cock nests in this copse to entice a mate.

At dusk one winter's afternoon, I startled three teal on this smallest pond and found a lone wing in the reeds. Next morning I returned to photograph it and check the feathers in my identification guide. It seemed it had belonged to an ill-fated woodcock.

When night falls, shadows leach into the wet meadow, formerly part of Rushmead, untethering place from name. Along the marshy edges, common rush stems blur and dissolve as the land trembles between dusk and dark. One evening, crouching beside my old friend, the meadow oak, I feel the ancient water-mead holding its breath. A pair of indistinct shapes move through the darkness on a desire line from fields to reeds, muntjac deer most likely, crossing to the pond to drink. Oak bark knuckles my back, its touch reassuringly solid. Cold meadow-breath brushes my cheek. Lichen against my wrist rasps like a cat's tongue. I think of the forests of lichen and moss high up in the oak, their textures raw-honed by the darkness. But I'm not foolhardy enough to climb by night, so I remain on solid ground. Ground that shudders beneath my feet as a train passes by on the Great Northern line. I breathe out the noise and glare of my day: the house clutter, the dissonance of family schedules, the need, the clamouring of a thousand thoughts. Alone under the oak, I am silence.

The wetlands are soothing at night. Though a black fox has been spotted on the reserve, the sighting sounds intriguing rather than ominous, and a friend's WhatsApp message about a big cat in the meadow (quickly followed by clarification that it's an enormous moggy not a lion) makes me laugh. Whatever animals might be out there, darkness promises solitary peace that daylight cannot provide. Watching the pond one afternoon from behind this hawthorn, I surprised a man smoking weed with my cheery greeting. I thought it wise to reveal myself before he walked into me. During Covid lockdown, I met another man here – always a lone man, never a woman – who wanted to show me his bird photos and came too close for comfort. When the year turned towards darkness and boundaries between worlds became porous, I walked this path alone and imagined I was pursued by an unearthly swarm of bees. No eldritch haunting, I realised when a drone buzzed into view and hovered above my head. Being watched by wrens, water rails, reed buntings and no doubt many other creatures going about their business unseen and unheard: that feels companionable. But being observed by an unknown drone controller gave me the Samhain shivers.

By late summer, heavy rain clouds are gathering. The chalk streams, reedbeds and water meadows are not the only local landscapes prone to unpredictable flooding. My internal topology makes me susceptible to inundation and the weather warning recently has been raised to amber, suggesting (according to the Met Office) increased likelihood of impacts which could potentially disrupt my plans. It is becoming harder by the day to ignore the debilitating effects of long-term fatigue and anxiety. I feel I spend more time in bed than out of it and the physical weakness that accompanies these bouts of exhaustion is becoming more severe. Worse still, my old nemeses – Fatigue and Anxiety – have called on a new accomplice – Pain – to complete the unholy trinity.

While we're holidaying on the Isle of Portland on the Dorset coast in August, my period begins and ends, but the accompanying pelvic pain persists. I assume it's just one of those things and wait for it to go, but weeks later I am still in pain and it's getting worse. Reading my journal or social media posts, you would think my summer was all sun and ice creams and adventure. My holiday prose shimmers with chalkhill blues and hummingbird hawk-moths; I skip through limestone quarries with small coppers and graylings, lie nose to petal with knapweed, wild carrot, eyebright and red clover, the grass warm under my belly. Ravens and wall brown butterflies pass by. I find sea lavender and golden samphire on the cliffs, and wonder if the rock pipits have started a second brood. My last swift of the year disappears across the English Channel. I bid it safe passage.

Back home, I write about summer walks and pond dipping with the kids. During a butterfly survey, I record the first wasp spider for the Bedfordshire reserve where Dad volunteers. She is hanging motionless in the centre of her orb web, waiting for a grasshopper, cricket or fly to blunder into her silken trap, or for a smaller male to arrive so she can mate with him, then eat him. We spend a day getting high on winged things at The Lodge in Sandy. The kids dart after hawkers and chase after darters. We track down a silver Y moth and find a buzzard's primary feather. I create a busy outdoor life for myself with the magic of words, but in truth it is a half-life. I am lying by omission, every second sentence written in invisible ink. I worry other people will not want to know the whole – the holey – me. So, as always, I conceal my illness and anxiety. I retreat into my head and sever connections with friends and family when severe fatigue returns, as it does with a vengeance in early September. No one visits. My inbox messages go unanswered. I am an old hand at lying low, concealing illness as carefully in life as I do on the page.

I'm not sleeping well, so I go back on sleeping tablets. And after years without episodes, I've started having seizures again, generally when I wake in the morning feeling desperately anxious. So far, Col has been with me and the children haven't been around. But I worry it's only a matter of time until I have one when they're present. At least I think I've worked out what they are. A couple of years ago, I came across an article on dissociative or functional seizures. The symptoms were identical to mine. It's thought these seizures can be caused by past trauma and can be subconsciously triggered by extreme emotion. They are not due to epilepsy, but the physical reactions are not within the person's control. I'm not unconscious while convulsing, but often it feels like a struggle to breathe. It's like being in an alternate reality, trapped inside my own head with no way to return to the world outside. It makes me feel horribly ashamed of my lack of emotional and physical self-control.

As well as the seizures, my energy feels like it is draining away. I feel faint when I walk. Life outside my bedroom seems many worlds away. Days pass in a blur of meals in bed, wobbly excursions to the loo, endless lonely hours drifting between sleep and despair. When I find the energy, I sit up and write, but pain and anxiety often intervene. Lying in bed, I look out at the television aerial across the street. Its reflector has horizontal wires like a stave in musical notation. As birds land and change places on the lines, they compose a flock of tunes. Collared doves are minims, the starlings, crotchets. Fat woodpigeons squat semibreves. Heavy rain washes the notes away. After the torrent, a chorus of starlings fly up to the aerial. They land, squabble and settle into the opening of 'This Old Man, He Played One'. I sing along with the birds in my head.

After weeks in bed and months of abdominal pain, I can no longer deny that I need help. I grudgingly admit to my doctor that I am not coping well with anxiety, fatigue and pain. She suggests an appointment with the Chronic Fatigue Syndrome Service. I decline. She refers me to the hospital and prescribes antidepressants. I put the gynaecology appointment in my diary and the pills at the back of the cupboard. Then I shut the door.

In October, I finally make it back to the wetlands. Progress is frustratingly slow. It feels like I've aged 20 years since my last visit. Stopping to rest on a bench, I reflect that walking at a pace slightly slower than your average snail gives me more time to notice the little things – a white passion flower making a late break for freedom over a back fence, spangle galls on a fallen oak leaf, a crocodilian log cruising low over the playing fields. Even the bench nurtures new life. A flush of tiny seedlings push through fissures in the damp wood. When I reach my favourite oak in the rush meadow, my wobbly pins start misbehaving and I realise I've come too far. Sitting in the grass, breathing air scented with water mint, I listen to the wind playing the reeds. Later, much later, a call for backup and Col drives to the meadow to give me a lift home. It has been a Sunday of small successes.

A few days later, it's Apple Day in the market square. I'm supposed to be helping launch a new nature network initiative to encourage local folk to support wildlife in their gardens. I want to be involved alongside the rest of our small group, but I'm still feeling pretty grim. Sitting on a chair beside our stand, my role is to talk to people about the wildlife they see in their gardens and encourage them to join our community nature network. We have a box of treasures: oak marble galls from the water meadows, ghostly dragonfly exuviae, the wasps' nest from the snicket, a collection of feathers, foliage excavated by leaf miners, and empty moth pupae. Traces and trappings of creatures that have since moved on. Apple Day is a friendly event, but this year all the people milling round the square frighten me. There are too many of them, too much colour and noise. I feel light-headed and hot. Panic rises, so I detach and watch the scene from outside myself. Like the show-and-tell collection, I have left my earthly trappings behind. As the action around me recedes, I wonder if I am going to have a seizure right here in the middle of the square. Fortunately, passing families come over to chat. I ask the children what they think lived in the empty nymph exoskeletons and what might have made the spherical galls. Their enthusiastic and wacky answers bring me back down to earth and remind me how much I enjoy talking to young people about the natural world.

One afternoon, Col finds me doubled-up over the kitchen floor. I'm supposed to be making dinner but the pain has ambushed me: my abdomen shoots fire and I can't think of anything but *When will it stop? Please make it stop.*

I'm glad *he* found me, not the kids. I try to hide away when the pain is bad so they won't worry. Occasionally, they find me in my bedroom curled over on all fours, some deep physical instinct inducing me to hunker down like I did in labour. I wish I could rise above my body and get on with life. I wish they didn't have to see me in pain or fret about me. I don't want the unpredictability that undermined my childhood to pass on to the next generation. I want to break that cycle.

Sometimes I wonder if I could detach from the pain and float away, like a magician's assistant severed by a merciful blade, my two halves existing independently of each other. But I lack the magic touch. However hard I try, my lower half remains stubbornly attached, my pain sensors in constant communication with my cortex. There are many ways of splitting oneself in two to dissociate from pain. This is one I've yet to learn.

In October half-term, we head off for a week on the Suffolk coast. I am still not right, and this is not the first time this year that the children have been on holiday and I've not been functional. It's rotten when I want to join in their activities but instead I'm forced to rest or curl up with the pain in bed on my own. One morning though, I find the energy to rise before dawn, fulfilling a promise to Helena to watch sunrise over the sea together. I pack my pockets with biscuits and we steal out of the cottage. A gust of wind flicks a long strand of hair across her eyes and I tuck it under her hat. We pick our way across the dunes, past the spot where we knelt yesterday marvelling at the tiny antlered leaves of buck's-horn plantain and stripping the remaining seeds from the yellow horned-poppy pods, scattering them across the sand on our way back to the cottage like a trail of botanical breadcrumbs.

At the top of the shingle ridge, the ground shifts under us and we slide, laughing, down the other side, running hand in hand to meet the sea. Strung-out lines of gulls fly south, barely discernible until they lift in silhouette above the horizon. The sun rises coral-pink over the sea and we play tag with the incoming tide, then scrunch up the strandline, scanning the berm for cast-off treasures – common whelk eggs, milky lozenges of sea glass, hagstones.

She soon gets bored of searching and starts a sand sculpture of a dragon. I find a couple of hagstones, but they are heavy and lopsided, nothing like the perfectly smooth specimen I found here earlier in the week. I'd never seen hagstones before this holiday, but this beach seems blessed with them, most with their holes packed full of tiny fragments of rock and other debris. When I spotted the warm brown pebble with its jammed hole on my first visit to the beach, I picked it up and put it in my pocket to leave my hands free to gather sea litter – tangles of orange fishing wire, a half-corroded glove, a mishmash of plastic bottles, lids and yoghurt pots.

Back at the cottage, I operated on the hagstone with a knife, freeing the hole and threading it with a piece of fluorescent green string from Jamie's yo-yo. Now the hagstone hangs down between my breasts like a talisman. When I hold its warm presence in a tight fist, it earths me. It reminds me how it feels to be standing in the waves, looking out to sea. Breathing air salted with freedom and hope. On our return home, I will slip it on a leather cord that once held a haematite pendant. I'm just borrowing the stone, I decide. For courage. I need its protection when anxiety threatens to drown me. One day, I hope I'll be able to find this strength within myself. One day, I will return it to the waves. But, for now, I am relying on the time-worn power of stone and sea.

I am sitting on a cantilevered willow branch beside the old watercress beds on a mild November afternoon, when the doctor's surgery sends a text asking me to book an appointment. Trying to keep calm, I ring and endure nearly half an hour of muzak that drowns out wren's song and flowing spring water. Finally, the receptionist answers and tells me my test results were abnormal. It seems I need to discuss them with the doctor. My heart sinks.

When the gynaecologist suggested an ultrasound a few weeks ago to investigate the cause of my chronic pelvic pain, I was grateful but apprehensive. My ability to cope with hospitals varies depending on how well I am managing my anxiety. Since Covid, it has been far worse, and I was concerned a scan might bring on a seizure.

I think back to our visit to the ultrasound department, Col and I discussing whether he should ask to come in or not. He's often told he can't accompany me, but most doctors relent and call him in when they're finding it tricky to get me to lie down or stay in the room. On this occasion he shouldn't even be in the waiting room according to the hospital's Covid rules and, anyway, I am determined to do this on my own.

The sonographer seems pleasant enough, though she is a woman of few words. A nurse stands in the corner, quiet and impassive. I am asked to confirm my details, which I manage with a nod, then remove trousers and pants and lie down. She dims the lights. We are silent. Without voices or light to anchor me, I feel myself start to slide inwards. All is elsewhere; the only activity in the room is the ultrasound probe moving gently inside me. My thigh muscles begin to harden, then my arms. I know where I'm heading and I don't want to go there, but this time I've brought protection. I reach for the leather cord around my neck and pull the hagstone out of my bra. I hold its warm presence, rub its familiarity against my thumb. Focus on this room. My body. My breath.

I tell myself it will soon be over.

When the sonographer finishes, I am still present, still in the room. I pull on my clothes and tie my shoes awkwardly. My only thought is to get out of there as quickly as possible. I slip out of the door and try not to run down the corridor. By the time I get to the car park, all I can think is that she said everything looked fine.

So now I've been told the results are abnormal, I don't know what to think. The receptionist cannot give me any further details and the first phone appointment is over a week away. I book it, then ring off. I am left alone in the meadow with my Schrödinger's womb. I try to puzzle out how a scan can be both normal and abnormal, but it remains an enigma. And this is not the first time I have stumbled over quantum theory in the water meadows. One afternoon last winter, I flushed four snipe that were hiding in the rushes. They zigzagged off, frightening the life out of me. Once I knew where they liked to forage, I kept away to avoid disturbing them. I'd take a roundabout route and wonder if they were feeding nearby. Without observing and almost certainly flushing them, I would never know. They were Schrödinger's snipe. Every time I visited, they were both present and not present. Fitting, I thought, for a landscape that embodies uncertainty: where paths moonlight as riverbeds, swamps drink themselves dry in high summer, and blackthorn volunteers engulf Yorkshire fog and cocksfoot grasses with their swift sprouting of bristly scrub.

I put my phone in my back pocket and look over at the path out. I am at the mercy of capricious landscapes inside and outside. If rampant blackthorn doesn't block the way or overflowing pools confound my sense of direction, the river will swamp the ford, preventing my escape. Fear floods in. I retreat. Consciousness shrinks to the dimensionless locus of pelvic pain that rumbles on inside.

I hear sirens. More sirens. Human voices and the rumble of machinery in the new building site adjacent to the water meadows. Beeping mechanical monsters reversing. Still more sirens, and now I am not sure if they are within or without. Alarm in the landscape; alarm in the body. We try to define paradoxical places and organs with our maps, units, axes and scans. But how can we observe the uncertain and record the amorphous?

To escape the sirens, I get to my feet and head to Shadwells Pool, noting the animal browns of the tussock sedges smouldering against willowherb stems greying into winter. Despite rotting vegetation all around, sedges hold life in their tints and highlights; they radiate a ginger heat. Looking across the spring-fed pool to the horizontal swathe of meadow, I realise I have transitioned from my one-dimensional world to two dimensions without noticing, and already I feel freer and less alarmed. Still sirens behind me, but only one. The sound no longer comes from within and without. The sensation of feet sinking in mud distracts me from the gnawing pain. I walk away from the pool and halt before a black puppet in the grass. Marinating in its own fluid, a liquid mole lies at my feet. Otherworldly up here in the light, its foreclaws look too powerful to be stilled by death. I imagine them in motion, digging. It takes me with it back to earth, burrowing into the third dimension. Down. Down. Vertical mole.

Above me, the beeping and rumbling has stilled. The contractors have finished for the evening, leaving only the gentle drone of traffic from the A505. As kestrel hunts, dusk falls over the sedges. Mole dreams of older lulls that settled over the Lammas meadows and springs at eventide. Cattle browse before lying down to sleep, small animals move through the grasses, gentle noises that rewind half a millennium or more, to a time before building sites, chemical pollution, over-extraction and global warming. When this chalk stream was still home to trout and eels, and water voles built their nests in lush sedge beds. Here beside Shadwells Pool, one metre down, five centuries in the past, I'm fully four-dimensional again, all pain and anxiety forgotten in the wonders of time and space.

After a December coppicing session, I walk home smelling of woodsmoke and sit at the piano to play and sing Mendelssohn's 'O for the Wings of a Dove' from Psalm 55. I am already missing the peace of the alder carr. The final couplet fills me with wild desire:

In the wilderness build me a nest,
And remain there forever at rest.

I want to build that nest. I turn to the landscape for salvation as my mental and physical health deteriorate. The phone appointment about the scan has revealed that my pain is likely caused by adenomyosis and I've been added to the gynaecology waiting list to see a consultant, but I have no idea how long it will be before I'm seen and whether I'll be offered more effective pain relief. In the meantime, my relationship with this place is both saving grace and snare. I burrow into the wetlands by night to escape the day. I tread on reeds that hiss like snakes. I build a bed of willow leaves and listen to the rustlings of the more-than-human world. I am watched by red eyes in the darkness. It feels easier to ground myself out here, to remain present, wrapped in the safety blanket of wild indifference. But fear and despair are waiting to claim me as soon as I leave. Though I have a greater insight into the reasons for my anxiety since revisiting my childhood, this new understanding has not made the emotions themselves any less agonising.

I cut myself a new hazel staff in the carr while coppicing, then prop it against a hawthorn while I have tea with the other volunteers and forget to take it home with me. When I return the day after Boxing Day, it is still leaning where I left it. Gripping the new pole firmly in my right hand, I thank the hawthorn and wonder if the May tree's protection will extend to me. Will the staff lead me, sure-footed, along the most treacherous of paths? Through fickle wetlands where what is solid becomes liquid, and what is hale sickens. Where fatigue floats beneath the surface, apt to flood its surroundings intermittently and unpredictably.

What if I were a chalk stream? Perhaps then I would go with the flow. I am, after all, over 50 per cent water. Less than half of me belongs to dry land. I, no, we (for surely water shares a collective consciousness) would rise from the springs that perforate this land...

from wellhead
    bubble tumble flow

above blue-sky
    gravel below

past stagnant ditch
   in ancient wood

bubble ripple
   roll and flood
song of grass
   and peewits call
bubble tumble
   rise and fall

above blue-sky
   gravel below
bubble ripple
   sing and flow

rill roll rush
   in pool we
p
     l
       u
         n
         g
         e

earth swallows all
down swallow hole

suckslurp
surgegush
we race

and rush
deeptime
darkflow
resurge
upthrow
as fast as spring
   we lightflow sing
bubble tumble
    speed and grow
above blue-sky
    gravel below

we meet ourselves
   in double flush
where ash greets riddy
    both brooks rush
past boggy carr
    where alders sup
we rise in ninesprings
    churning up
from mud pools
    bubble tumble sing
join purwell river
    shadwells spring

then into flooded meadows seep
    where herons hunt
and orchids sleep
    we gain the ford
and gather speed

by anchor millstream burymead
we greet the hiz
   and northwards go
bubble tumble
   sing and flow
above blue-sky
   gravel below

We are giddy and more than a little relieved to climb out of the waters and bid the chalk stream farewell as it flows into Bedfordshire. Shaking like a dog, we free ourselves from every last drop of shared consciousness and reclaim the singular first-person pronoun. After springs, swallow holes, winterbournes and water meadows, I need to find some dry land.

When I get home from the alder carr, I prop my staff behind the door in the shed. My last staff was recommissioned as a chicken perch and I don't want to lose another. Hazel is the dowsing tree. Rod of the water witcher. I'll need its charms to gain safe passage through the fluid landscapes that lie ahead.

By February, I'm brittle with anxiety. Sleep is elusive. Nights cramped with pain; dreams troubled by portents I can't decode.

I refuse to take my mum to her medical appointments.
I watch someone drown in the icy sea.
I sit in a theatre looking out over bare shoulders and realise everyone in the auditorium apart from me is naked.

I steal money to buy a lawnmower.
I start lactating again.

Though April brings the first kingcups, cuckooflowers and orange-tip butterflies, and Daddy Blackbird is feeding his chicks in their honeysuckle nest above our patio windows, I can't shake the fear. At times it is so acute I cannot bear to speak to anyone. Lying in bed during the day, I hear car doors slam outside. Every bang strikes me in the chest. They are coming for me. I don't know who they are, but they are surely coming.

One night when the despair is almost unbearable, I hear the sedge pool calling. I am lying on my side in bed, left cheek damp against the pillow in a wetland of my own making. I'm in deep, drowning in the mire of my mind, when I hear the call from that warm, animal pool. It wants me. It is waiting. I imagine lowering my body into water, an inch-by-inch submission. The ultimate immersion in nature. Sinking into this thought, I fall asleep. In the morning when I wake, I put the pool out of my mind.

But I'm running out of fight. I'm tired. Tired of anxiety. Tired of tiredness. So very tired of being me. Every day I feel anxiety stirring... spreading. Why does it grow? Why its desire to consume and command? What will be left behind when I have served my purpose?

A host. A husk. Mere end matter.

This is how I feel when fear takes hold. When it fills me so entirely that any other thoughts seem impossible. When paranoia seizes me, twisting my guts, wringing shame from every pore. This is how it feels when I hear the moaning and know the sounds come from my chest, my throat, my pain. This is how I wake, drenched in sweat, jerking, thrashing. A body out of control.

Anxiety is a parasite: it feeds on emotions. As it gorges and grows strong, I become weak, in thrall to the belief that I am culpable beyond forgiveness. Of what, I'm not always sure, but whatever it is, I know I deserve hatred and humiliation. I watch myself cower and writhe. I know I've lost control and I despise this parasitised self.

One morning it crushes me as soon as I wake, before I've even time to register the room, the time, the light. I can't move for the noise of it in my head, all the things I must achieve today, my feelings of inadequacy and fear. I feel my biceps tighten. Distress spreads. Up. Down. Neck. Thighs. All warped. Head crooked on the pillow. Arms and legs contorted. I am a china doll, dropped and broken. I hear Col somewhere near, talking to me, encouraging me to stay in the room. I've not started convulsing, so I think perhaps I can beat this.

"What can you see?" he asks. "Five things you can see..." I can't answer. Nothing. I see nothing. He tries again. "What can you hear?" The window is open. Outside there's a tinkling. No sight, but I can hear music in the garden.

"Goldfinch," I say, quietly, thickly, like it's the first word I've ever spoken. Goldfinch. Then the words get easier. My breathing. A car. I've stopped listening inside and found the world outside my head. The world of the goldfinch. And once I start to think about birds, my leg and arm muscles unclench, my neck relaxes. I'm lying in bed again, on a spring morning, with a day ahead of me that I know I'll get through, somehow.

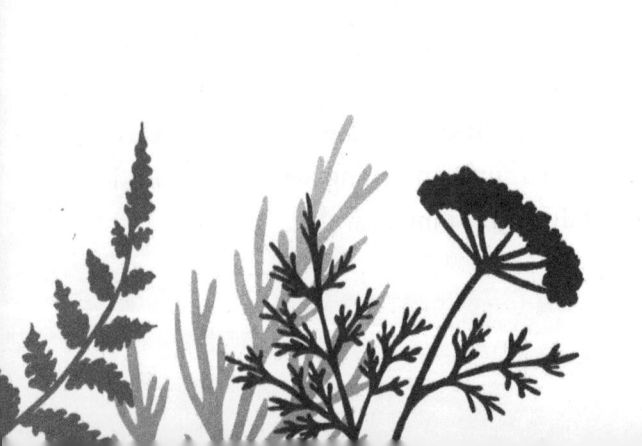

Chalkbones

Summer comes round and I'm back in bed again. Propped up against the pillows, talking to my counsellor over Zoom. Or rather, listening to the space she has left for me, wondering how I might fill it with words. I don't remember the last time I felt this low, this exhausted and frightened. So hollow I'm not sure I care much about anything anymore. I feel old ghosts stirring. I don't know how much longer I can keep them penned in.

I look away from the screen. Stare out of the bedroom window. Eye contact is not exactly my strong point and, besides, the sycamore is waving at me. Tossing its top branches in a breeze whose rousing touch I'd like to feel on my skin. In bed, I inhale. Stale air. Sour with sweat.

The pause tips over. Into. Agony. An accusing silence, jeering. Louder even than the tinnitus that stings and sings in my ears. "FILL ME," it mocks.

"So empty there are no words?"
"Pain so shameful you cannot admit it aloud?"
"Cat got your tongue?"

It's hard to ignore the accusations. My volume control is turned up so loud, I'm shattered by the white noise of scorn. But out there, the wind is free. It blows me a gift...

... tumbling out of the sky like it's fallen from heaven. Down behind my neighbours' house, all forked tail and retracted wings, plunging. Bigger than my pain. I sit up and lean across the pillows to catch the red kite as it rises and passes the window, so close it almost fills the panes. It's not finished. I want to know what's caught its eye, what it covets so much that it comes round again, drops again. Then again. Five times in all. When it pulls up from the final plunge, circles the rooftops and disappears, I've no idea if it's off for a lap of honour or to find its next meal.

As the drama unfolds, closer to the window than I have ever seen this huge raptor before, I'm narrating to my counsellor. I can't help myself. I want her to see it too. To know what a privilege it is to witness this behaviour and feel the bird so nearby. She is watching me closely. I know she is, because I'm meeting her eye now, sharing my pleasure that something unexpectedly good has just happened. And once I start talking, it is like a dam breaking. I tell her how important the birds outside my window are on the days I can't get out of bed. I tell her about my birthday heron – the long-legged fish-spearing thunderbolt that brings me many happy returns. How rarely we see herons on the neighbours' rooftop, only three or four times a year, but every winter for three years a heron has been waiting, poised impossibly tall when I've opened the curtains on my birthday morning. So reliable that last time my daughter was expecting it and came haring in to wake me. "Your birthday heron's here Mummy, it's here."

My counsellor tells me how my face changes when I talk about birds. How they bring me alive. I could go on to explain how, one year, the children read to the rooftop heron out of the window from Robert Macfarlane and Jackie Morris's spellbinding *The Lost Words*, replacing 'weir' with 'window', so in our version the bird rests 'still still at windowsill'. Or how, on bad days, I measure the hours by swift flight and kite flight. How I listen as robin song becomes greenfinch, then blackbird, goldfinch and dunnock. How sparrows bicker beneath the bathroom window and wood pigeons roll past, bobbing gently on cooing waves. But instead, I find myself talking about pain and dizziness. The fact that my legs won't hold me, and all I want to do is sleep, except at night. About the way I am sure I'd rattle if someone shook me, a jangle of sleeping pills, painkillers and vitamins. I talk about anxiety and fear. I tell her how afraid I am that somewhere inside I am rotten, callous, broken and soon someone will find me out. I tell her how I pick over the words I say and write, how I worry them ragged to find evidence of my iniquity. I tell her how hard I am finding it right now, how tired I am of fighting, how close I am to despair. She asks a question no one has dared ask me before. I'm not sure I can answer. But with the unspoken spoken, I feel a little lighter. A little less ashamed. Still sad, still stale. The air still still at windowsill. And yet I've remembered there *is* a life outside. Perhaps tomorrow I will sit in the garden for a few minutes. Or if not tomorrow, then sometime soon. And I think I know now what the red kite came down for. And I think it carried a little of it away.

John Clare, the Northamptonshire poet, was born on 13 July 1793. Every year on the weekend closest to his birthdate, a festival is held in the village of Helpston, where Clare lived until he was 38. We first attended four years ago after I discovered my great-great-great-great-grandparents, John and Mary Howsden, had lived in the same house as John and Martha Clare in the early nineteenth century. Each family had a one-up one-down tenancy in a shared cottage, and both Mary and Martha had nine children within a 17-year period, 14 of whom (seven in each family) survived to adulthood. The 1826 Helpston Parish Register lists the birth of Alice Howsden, fifth child of Mary and John the shepherd, on the same page as the birth of John Clare, fifth child of Martha and John the poet.

I have met some lovely people in Helpston, including Peter Wordsworth, a villager whose farming family employed my great-great-great-uncle, William Patrick, as a horseman. I treasure a picture Peter gave me of William with one of Peter's family's horses in 1921, when William was 73. He died later the same year after being severely burned while trying to extinguish a hedge fire. After his death, his wife, Eliza Patrick (one of John and Mary Howsden's granddaughters), moved into the almshouses in the village, where my granny met her in 1928. I've enjoyed going back to my literary roots, researching the lives of some of Clare's contemporaries in the village, including my own family, and writing up my research for the *John Clare Society Journal*.

The 2022 John Clare Festival is the first since Covid. There will be readings and lectures and folk music. I want to play with my great-great-great-grandfather Henry (oldest son of John and Mary) in the garden at Clare Cottage where he likely took his first steps, holding his hand as he toddles through the hollyhocks, chasing him round and round the apple tree. And I'd like to meet up with members of the living I've not seen for a while too.

But July has not been a good month. I seem to be losing contact with my legs. Door frames, walls and bannisters scaffold my slow journeys around the house. I haven't made it to the reedbeds for weeks. One day I walk a matter of metres to the end of the road to visit the traveller's joy. The world swims in and out of focus as if I'm opening my eyes underwater. Wild clematis floats through the hedge in flagrant profusion, thousands of ivory stamens splayed like sea anemone tentacles. The flowers are blurry with bees. I sit on our road sign for a while to recover, then rise and drift dizzily downstream towards the house. My agency over life seems to be draining away by the day.

Col and the kids pack the car and we make it to Helpston, but my legs refuse to take my weight. Leaning heavily on Col's arm, I walk to the church for the festival talks. While I listen, he takes the kids round the village. Afterwards, I wait in my seat to be collected. It is impossible to pretend I'm okay, but no one asks what's up, and I'm relieved not to have to explain myself. I've no clue why I was able to walk unaided a few weeks ago, yet now I must cling to Col's arm to stop myself collapsing. In the past I'd have hidden away at home, but this is the second time this year I've chosen to attend an event where I knew my illness would be obvious to other people.

The first was in May when I led a writing workshop for the Sussex Wildlife Trust during ME/CFS Awareness Week. I'd been asked to contribute to *Moving Mountains*, an anthology of nature writing by authors living with chronic illness and physical disability. The idea terrified me. I felt unworthy to be included alongside people who, without doubt, had far harder challenges to overcome than I do. Writing also involved committing that part of myself to paper that I had, so far, refused to own. But I knew that eliding the days when I was unable to get out of bed simply perpetuated the myth that worthwhile encounters with the natural world happen only to wild people in wild places. I engage with the natural world differently when I am ill – through windows, in books and my imagination, through slow observation – and I was starting to realise these times were an important part of my personal story.

I agreed to write a piece, hoping it might help address the way severe fatigue can fall through the gaps in nature writing, lost in elisions around which the story softly folds and closes. Perhaps, I thought, by opening the windows and stepping out of the shadows, I'd feel more able to embrace the still moments, to share the view from my bed of the sycamore in the shaft between the houses shaking autumn loose, and the crows dancing, slowly, on the rooftops.

I led the writing workshop on Zoom as part of a project connected to the anthology. We focused on different ways to find inspiration in nature when circumstances restrict you to slow walks or watching wildlife from the window. It was the first time I'd given a talk while identifying as a writer with a chronic illness. The workshop went smoothly, apart from an impromptu star turn by one of our Orpington bantams. Having laid an egg halfway through the session, Burnet decided to celebrate her achievement with an ear-piercing coloratura, chicken-style. Her operatic interruption threw my concentration for a minute. Then I had to laugh. How many times have I broken the two fundamental rules of show business: never work with children or animals? But what better way to ensure that life is never ever boring?

Best of all, I felt that buzz which arises spontaneously from the joy of sharing information that is just too good to keep to yourself. The feedback was warm and enthusiastic. It was lovely to think I might have encouraged others to spend a little time appreciating a self-sown flower in a pavement crack or a party of swifts tearing past the window, and I hoped each noticing might give them as much pleasure as it does me.

In the third week of July, temperatures soar to 40 degrees Celsius in parts of the UK for the first time since records began 350 years ago. We've had only 11 per cent of the normal monthly rainfall in Hertfordshire, and many areas in the South have had far less. People, plants, wildlife and chalk streams are all suffering. The lawn shrivels, but my tiny wildflower patch attracts the goldfinches. Their ability to perch on knapweed and yarrow seed heads, bending them almost to the ground without breaking a single stem, is a lesson in weights and balances, and their irrepressible bounce is a tonic to the jaded observer. Behind the wildflowers, the plum harvest lies withered on the ground like so many shrunken heads. Only the greengages remain hanging: a mash-up of sorry flesh and wasps' waggling arses.

Despite the drought, I am struggling to keep my head above water. Every time my energy levels ebb, anxiety takes possession and I forget how to be in the world. I know I've been thrown a lifeline – it's been over six months since the doctor prescribed antidepressants for anxiety and panic attacks – but I am too afraid to grab it. Though I cannot see the tablets on the top shelf of the cupboard, I know they are there. I have several friends who take them, and they've all been supportive, some telling me how they wished they had started their own treatment earlier. I can see they've made sensible decisions, but taking pills myself feels like accepting help for which I do not qualify.

The Nic writing this book can see there is a problem. She's been writing it for months now, so it is an old story as far as she's concerned. With a bit of narrative distance, the pattern is irrefutable. Writing Nic takes risks. She wants to try antidepressants to see if they make life any kinder. The packet burns on the back shelf of her mind. What if the pills contain peace rather than fear? What if owning up to anxiety and accepting treatment is a way forward, not a cop-out?

She could take just one tablet. Tell no one. But writing Nic is not in charge in the kitchen and the packet remains unopened. It is hard to break the habit of more than one lifetime. And all the while she is ramping through the book, climbing through childhood and dragging herself into adolescence, remembering what it felt like to teach and hold bairns in her arms, how a new diet changed her and how she fell in love with the local landscape. Now she is approaching herself, her present – and she wants to know what happens next. Does she grasp her courage and weather the first few weeks of antidepressants, which can, apparently, make you feel worse? Come out the other side with an emerging sense of what it feels like to temper her anxiety? Or does she reject the help and keep going as always, managing her emotions as best she can? Neither of them knows. But they will arrive at the 'now' very soon and there will be a reckoning to face if they want to carry on.

Like me, Jamie has always been an avid reader. When he starts to read books for young adults, I grab the chance to revisit stories I loved as a child and discover new authors. Much as I did, he wanders through fantasy worlds, inhabiting them for weeks at a time. He devours our Terry Pratchett collection, so we buy him *The Wee Free Men*, the first of a sequence of Discworld novels about Tiffany Aching, a nine-year-old soon-to-be witch-in-training who lives in the chalk hills. Pratchett's witch stories are full of powerful female characters, and this series, with its straight-talking, boot-wearing heroine, is no exception.

One day as Tiffany lies by the river tickling trout, she hears a susurrus. The air fizzes. The water bubbles. Tiffany reads the signs and hastens back from the edge, just before Jenny Green-Teeth, a river-monster from *The Goode Childe's Booke of Faerie Tales*, jumps out of the water and attempts to grab her. Back home, Tiffany studies the creature in Granny Aching's copy of the book and returns to dispatch it quickly and efficiently with a frying pan, using her younger brother as bait. Later in the day, she visits a band of travelling teachers and meets Miss Tick, a witch who, being very sensitive to geology, does not believe it is possible to do magic on chalk. Witches need hard rocks like granite or basalt, but Tiffany is tough and sharp despite living above the soft tiny bones of billions and billions of sea creatures. She is an anomaly. A *chalk* witch.

I see a little of myself in Tiffany. Her liking for the taste of words, the way fairy tales come alive around her. We both have shepherding ancestors. I had a granny who used old words, left me her wildflower books and taught me about the nature of the hills. People tend to leave me alone too. And, like Tiffany, I live on the chalk.

Although I was not born here, I am a sedimentary lass at heart. My geologic timescale chart shows moulding by sandstone, mudstone and siltstone, then maturation on the chalk:

Year	Place	Geology	Period	Approx. Date (Ma)
1975–83	Nuneaton	Sandstone	Cambrian	500
1983–93	Cuddington	Bollin Mudstone	Triassic	240–50
1993–2003	Durham	Mudstone/ Siltstone/ Sandstone	Carboniferous	300
2003–	Hitchin	Chalk	Cretaceous	90–100

I've tried excavating those first three decades for memories of what lay beneath my feet, but not much has been preserved. A few scratchings with sticks in sandy garden soils; a primary school visit to the salt museum in Northwich to learn about the Triassic salt beds that underlie the Cheshire basin; vague recollections of singing Verdi's 'Dies Irae' and feeling our voices reverberate off the sandstone vaults of Durham Cathedral, itself high on a great sandstone bluff – the dun holme or 'hill island' after which the city was named – formed by the winding of the River Wear. Grainy recollections at best. I was too busy forging my identity and dreaming of the future. Too young to feel the deep, deep time beneath me. But now I feel it. After two decades settling in Hertfordshire at the north-easternmost edge of the Chilterns, like the sedimentary rock of the Cretaceous period, I feel calcareous through every cross section.

And what about you, I wonder, looking at the chalk hill rising from my palm. Will you help me connect with the land? Ever since I found you on the internet, I've been excavating your secret history. *Conulus*, they call you, but that's a dead name. I refuse to invoke your epitaph. Leave that for inscriptions on museum labels and faded photographic plates. I prefer to whisper folk names to you: "My fairy's nightcap, my thunderstone, my shepherd's crown." Names that conjure your lifeform. Names that quicken your domed nub, a microcosmic echo of the Benslow chalk knoll across the road where railway lines parted the soft hill and unearthed a Cretaceous tomb.

You were there when the land began. While the calcareous ooze accumulated, you waited in your stronghold on the shallow shelf seabed. As you fed, crawling across the sea floor on your tube feet, the sediment stirred to life and danced like motes of dust rising in a warm room.

You must have been formidable in your day. Your shell was made of calcium carbonate plates that protected your internal organs housed within rather like the coiled tubes and consoles of that other veteran time-traveller, the TARDIS. Your spines, attached to the plates by ball-and-socket joints, may have offered some protection from the shadows that passed between you and the sun. Did you use them to wedge yourself in cracks and crevices when the shell-crushing *Ptychodus* shark cruised past on the hunt for bivalves and crustaceans to grind between its huge ridged teeth?

You, at least, escaped death by grinding. I can testify to that for here you are, tapering up from my palm like a conical growth. Your pentamerous symmetry rising to meet me, your radial bands (from which your tube feet protrude) converging in a five-pointed star at your apex. You have acclimatised to my hand, so I touch my lips to your milky-grey underside as though your mouth is a child's forehead. Is there a kindling within, a spark of ghost-life? Do you have flint at your heart? No, I think not. Your mouth is cool against mine and your lithic skin feels granular. Like me, I suspect you are now chalk through and through.

Sea urchins like you – now represented by your fossilised remains – were once commonplace in the warm, shallow shelf seas of the late Cretaceous epoch. When the railway cutting near my house was excavated during the Victorian period, the fossils found in the cliff face became an important resource for understanding the chalk sequence in southern England. They included the echinoderm *Conulus subrotundus* along with bivalves, brachiopods and sharks.

Many specimens are now stored in the headquarters of the British Geological Survey at Keyworth in Nottinghamshire. But with no access to these local fossils when I start exploring the chalk during Covid lockdowns, I search instead for *Conulus* online. I want to touch the past, to weigh the origins of the land in my hand. The shepherd's crown I choose is from Kent rather than Hertfordshire, but feeling its chalky form on my palm gives me the physical and emotional conduit I'm looking for.

I delve into local museum archives and trawl through geological journals. I read about a Watford Natural History Society field trip on a warm June afternoon in 1877. Absorbed in the account, I can almost believe I'm standing beside William and Alfred Ransom in the chalk pit across the road at Hitchin railway station, listening to renowned archaeologist and geologist Sir John Evans discussing the different layers of chalk and the beds of clay and gravel that overlie them, which he believes to have been formed in the glacial period. Next, I travel back on a field trip to the same chalk pit, this time in 1896 with Hitchin farmer and geologist William Hill, who, along with fellow geologist Alfred John Jukes-Browne, first described the railway site in detail a decade earlier. On this expedition, Hill points out fossilised bivalves and explains that the Melbourn Rock at the base of the Middle Chalk is where a shark tooth from *Ptychodus mammillaris* was discovered.

The more I learn about the bedrock beneath me, the more I identify with this place I've come to think of as home. Though I'd like to be flint like my hagstone – hard, durable, a fire starter – in reality, I'm all chalk: a bit soft, immersed in the past, an inextricable affinity with the sea. All those tiny flakes of life and death accreting on the seabed over millions of years. The landform created from their recycled calcium enduring for aeons. When Tiffany Aching calls on the power of the hills in her fight with the Queen of the Fairies at the end of *The Wee Free Men*, she is drawn down through layers of time to the very heart of the chalk. She hears her own voice in her head telling her the land is in her bones and, when she draws on this inner force, on the power of stars and years, of space and time, nothing, no one, can stand against her.

But I'm no witch-in-training. Though I layer up my thermals when out in the field, having never ridden a broomstick, I've not yet felt the need to don three pairs of pants. It has never occurred to me to wield kitchenware against the demons of my imagination. And I don't know how to call on the power of the land. When water rises and inundation threatens, the ground beneath me feels frangible, ravaged with holes. Where is the strength in chalk – in me?

"Are you feeling brave?" the consultant asks, looking at me over his mask.

It has been nearly a year since my abnormal ultrasound revealed I had adenomyosis and eight months since I was advised to have a Mirena coil fitted to alleviate my chronic pain. It sounded simple when the consultant explained the process – a quick trip to my local sexual health clinic to have an IUD that would release tiny amounts of progesterone to help with the bleeding and reduce the pain.

But the sexual health clinic refused to see me because I wanted pain relief rather than contraception, so I tried the doctor's. It took over a month to arrange a phone appointment with the practice specialist, who agreed to fit one a few weeks later. I went to the first fitting by myself. An unwise decision, as it turned out. I thought, given the appointment was at the doctor's rather than the hospital, and with a female GP, I'd be able to handle it. But I could feel myself dissociating almost immediately. I stopped making eye contact. My answers became monosyllabic. Almost inaudible. When the doctor asked if I wanted her to fit it, I nodded. She hesitated, weighing me up. I think it was my history of seizures that decided it. I left with a prescription for beta blockers to help control my anxiety. At the bottom of the prescription, she had written an instruction for next time: 'Bring your husband'.

For the second appointment I took painkillers, beta blockers and Col. This time the doctor got as far as the fitting, setting up and measuring my uterus before problems set in. I was working hard to manage my anxiety and pain, holding the hagstone in a tight fist. When she started to insert the Mirena, it felt like the end was in sight. Then my cervix decided enough was enough. It closed and refused further entry. In the end there was no alternative but to withdraw the coil, bent and defeated. Cervix 1: Mirena 0. The doctor referred me back to the hospital.

Months later, with rising pain levels and little in the way of pain relief, I'd still had no word of an appointment, just a letter explaining that the gynaecology department might refer me back to my doctor as their waiting list had become unfeasibly long. Eventually I contacted the hospital to ask how such a simple procedure, one that could potentially save me from distressing pain, could be so hard to arrange. Several phone calls later they found a last-minute cancellation. I was booked in for the following day.

So, when the consultant asks me if I'm feeling brave, I stare at him, considering. I'm not sure what he wants me to say. I think he means "This is going to hurt. Are you going to make a fuss?" Given I am already in pain, even though I'm on paracetamol and codeine, I have no idea how much more I'll be able to take before I crack.

"Um, I'm not sure," I say. "But I want it in." He calls the nurse and asks for a coil. She tells him they don't have any. There is a puzzled silence. I am in a gynaecology department in a large modern hospital. I have finally managed to see a consultant after nine months of waiting for the procedure that could help control my chronic pain, and they don't even have a fucking coil.

He writes a prescription and hands it to me. "Take this to the hospital pharmacy," he says, "and see if they have any." I trot downstairs dutifully and give it to the pharmacist, who tells me they can't prescribe coils because gynaecology dispenses them. I wonder if Kafka is hiding in the shampoo aisle.

Back upstairs, I go to the main desk and ask if I can speak to the consultant again. The receptionist takes exception to my unreasonable request. Can't I see, she says, that this is antenatal reception, not gynaecology? There's a sign. She points. I ask who I should talk to. She says she has no idea. By this point, I'm definitely not feeling brave. I can feel the tears rolling down inside my mask.

Someone goes to find the consultant, and he comes out looking harried. "Ring my secretary and I'll try to fit you in next week," he says. We head off home. I don't have much faith in his plan. Perhaps I will be able to persuade the switchboard to give me his secretary's number (he can't remember it) and maybe they'll give me another appointment. It's even possible they might have a coil to hand this time. But I suspect Kafka will pop up again, somewhere along the way.

After numerous phone calls to three different hospitals, I have the coil fitted late one afternoon in the maternity unit where I gave birth to my children. Walking down the long corridor that we last took the day before Helena's birth evokes poignant feelings of déjà vu. The adenomyosis pain I feel today is not dissimilar to early labour cramps. But now, 13 years after I became a mother, I am here in search of pain relief which will tide me over until the menopause. Having visited the unit many times when my fertility was upfront and celebrated, I am now waiting for its power to wane, after which the hormone-induced pain will hopefully disappear.

This time the procedure is straightforward and successful. Despite asking how brave I'm feeling every time he meets me, the consultant is kind and gentle. I am back home within the hour, relieved that my nine-month wait is over. Next day, strong cramping kicks in and I check the internet to find out when the longed-for pain relief might start. Different adenomyosis websites give different timings: three to six months, a year or more, or possibly not at all. I am devastated. Naïvely, I thought it would work within the first few days. Despite all my research, I forgot to check this vital fact, and at no point during the whole absurdist drama did either the doctor or consultant think it important enough to mention.

Our house is filled with the cacophonous squawking of waterfowl and other pondlife. Col and Helena have started rehearsing *Honk!* – a musical based on the story of *The Ugly Duckling*. Once casting is over, it appears I am sharing the house with a dancing moorhen, a froglet, a singing fish and a raving tomcat, the villain of the piece. Fairy-tale wildlife assuming human form. While they frolic and footle and hunt around the pond, I lie high and dry in my bedroom wondering if I will ever be well enough to take part in another show. My saloon-dancing days in *Calamity Jane* seem a lifetime ago.

September and October are the worst months yet. Work is busy. I push on with writing, editing and research. I'm booked to give a talk on wildlife gardening to an allotment society in mid-September. I don't want to leave them in the lurch, so I get out of bed to attend, though my dodgy balance means Col has to drive me to the venue. I miss the choir concert for the third term running and send my apologies for the remaining Wildlife Trust sessions of the year. At a parents' event I really want to attend, dizziness swamps me and I have to sit it out. Staff kindly bring me a cup of tea and a banana. Once home, my body decides it is done.

Despite my dismay at another bout of exhaustion so soon after the last, I am determined not to withdraw this time. I try to lie lightly with the sense my energy limitations are faked or simply the result of a lack of determination. The unpredictable nature of chronic illness is as inexplicable to me as it is to my friends and family. Like an intermittent fault on a car, fatigue chooses its own time to strike. This does not, unfortunately, make it any less real. But I am done with self-doubt. Done with ignoring and pretending. This is who I am and this is what my body is – sometimes capable of functioning normally for weeks at a time, sometimes not. I am determined to accept that long-term fatigue does not make me less than. It is simply part of the whole me.

And other things are changing too. Little by little, I'm daring to discuss my illness with family members and a friend or two. I tell them how pissed off I am living on hold, without the energy to read or get out of bed or look after my children. How much I yearn to go to the meadow now the evenings are drawing in. How I miss the sighing of the reeds and the subtle changes taking place without me in the alder carr. Taking a deep breath, I post on social media about how difficult I am finding it to cope – the cancelled activities, not being able to get outside, worrying that life is leaving me behind, endless waiting for hospital appointments, my concerns about the effect my illness is having on my kids. The response from friends, both online and off, is kind and understanding. Almost imperceptibly, I've started letting people in.

I talk to the kids about how these times are just another part of life, and encourage myself not to feel ashamed when I am unable to get up with them in the mornings. Hearing an internal voice that supports and cherishes me is a powerful new experience. It gives me a sense of resolve. We turn my room into a communal space and share time together in bed until I am ready for the next nap. Childhood taught me chronic illness was self-indulgent and shameful. I intend to break that cycle. It is not a belief I want my children subconsciously absorbing. I am determined to be proud of who I am, in bed and out of it.

I probably don't pay as much attention as I should to the mineral content of my food. But living in a hard water area makes it difficult to ignore the effect of mineral deposits in the water, especially the limescale that cakes the intestines of our appliances, sometimes causing them to grind to a premature halt. Around two thirds of Hertfordshire's water supply is abstracted from the chalk aquifer that underlies the county. Having fallen as rain, water filters through the permeable ground dissolving calcium and magnesium in the chalk as it makes its way through the aquifer, before eventually returning to the surface via natural springs or boreholes. By the time it reaches the taps, our water has one of the highest levels of calcium and magnesium in the UK, at 298 parts per million.

But the chalk beneath my feet is also testament to the protective power of calcium carbonate. As one of the most abundant minerals in seawater, calcium is readily absorbed by marine organisms such as echinoderms. The calcium is combined with carbonate ions to form crystals of calcium carbonate in a process called biogenic calcification. These crystals are then used to form plates, shells and skeletons. Coccolithophores – the main component of the Chalk – are single-celled algae surrounded with calcite plates that are thought to have several possible functions, including protecting them from being eaten. Echinoderms create an endoskeleton of interlocking calcium carbonate plates, often referred to as a shell or test, which provides support, structure and protection, and molluscs form external calcified shells. Like aquatic molluscs, land snails can absorb calcium from water, although they also ingest the mineral from the surrounding environment for processes such as shell growth and repair, and egg production. Some species eat leaves and decaying wood, or rasp on bones, rocks such as limestone, calcareous soils and other snails' shells to obtain calcium. Not all snails require calcium-rich habitats, but populations are more diverse and abundant on soils with a high pH like mine.

I've come across many species of snail on the chalky escarpments and in the wetlands, from heath snails curled up in windblown pasqueflower blooms to great pond snails in the reedbeds, their empty shells discarded in the mud, perhaps by foraging water shrews. But, during our 20 years living on chalk, we've met only one snail who became a part of the family. I spotted it one day down the side of the newly constructed raised beds about a year after we'd moved house, an alabaster-whorled centurion surrounded by a legion of bronze-uniformed garden snails. It was the biggest gastropod I'd ever seen, measuring a colossal (in snail terms) 4 centimetres. Only one land snail reaches these epic proportions in the UK: the Roman, or edible, snail, and as a calcicole or chalk-dweller, it is restricted to calcareous areas such as the chalky grasslands of the Chilterns. Thought to have been introduced by the Romans, these snails can live for a decade or more. The raised lip at the mouth of this snail's shell suggested it was a sexually mature adult, and the pale shell colour also indicated an older snail, as they lose the organic brown layer which protects the shell as they age. In his paper on his 1884 excavation of what he believed to be a Roman villa near Purwell Ninesprings, William Ransom (an extremely knowledgeable archaeologist alongside his other specialisms) speculated about the Roman habit of breeding edible snails and dormice near their villas. He quoted Marcus Terentius Varro, a famed Roman scholar, who proposed:

A proper place in the open air is to be provided to preserve snails, which you must compass all around with water, that you may find those you put there to breed, as well as their young ones. I say they are to be encompassed by water, that they may have no opportunity of escaping.

Could this snail's ancestors have returned to the wild, perhaps when the site was abandoned by the Romans, and established a population on my patch? A colony which endured unnoticed for nearly two millennia until the final survivor of a species which rarely moves more than 50 metres in its lifetime found itself without companions in our suburban garden? I know there are other isolated Roman snail communities elsewhere in Hertfordshire (one of which has been there for 300 years), but I have never seen or heard of a local population, so the origins of our garden giant remain an enigma. I guess it's always possible it was just an escaped pet; we'll never know.

Whatever the reason for Roman's presence in the garden, we were excited by our discovery. We sent a photograph of the snail posing beside a 30-centimetre ruler to The Conchological Society. When no reply was forthcoming, we looked out for Roman, a protected species, as best we could. We'd check when we went outside, taking care not to crush the snail underfoot when it embarked on a slow march across the lawn on damp days en route to the lettuce patch. The large pale shell contrasted with both foliage and soil, so Roman was never hard to find, unless it was time for hibernation. Then it would withdraw to a corner of the garden (one year I found it hibernating with its legion of molluscular mates behind the fruit cage) and produce a calcium carbonate lid called an epiphragm to close off the shell mouth, which remained in place until it returned to an active state in spring.

Once Roman had emerged, famished, the race to consume the contents of the vegetable beds to regain the weight loss sustained over winter began. Spring and summer sightings of the mighty mollusc crossing the lawn and munching on our lettuces continued for several years, until one spring, Roman failed to reappear. The sadness we felt at its absence was a measure of how much this individual snail had come to mean to us. A few weeks later I found the empty shell in the undergrowth by the shed, a chalky-white exoskeleton returned to the calcareous land from which it came.

Although dissimilar anatomically, humans share some of the same mineral requirements as both echinoderms and molluscs, and we, too, can absorb calcium from water and use it in our bodies. As any primary school child could tell you, we need calcium for maintaining healthy bones and teeth. Especially me. As a coeliac, I need to ingest more calcium every day than non-coeliacs. Studies have found evidence of reduced bone mineral density in up to 75 per cent of coeliacs when they are diagnosed, and it's thought the risk of osteoporosis may be higher in those who have a late or delayed diagnosis as an adult. Calcium can't be produced by biological processes, so an animal's diet – whether it be sea urchins absorbing calcium ions from seawater, snails rasping on limestone or Popeye scoffing spinach – is the only way to access this vital nutrient.

As I drink my mug of tea, a thin wafer settles on my tongue. Tasteless, brittle, easily punctured between my canines, it shatters into chalky fragments that wedge themselves in my molars. I extract the soft lumps with the tip of my tongue and, when I swallow, I'm ingesting time. Consuming rock, reforming bone and shell, recycling lifeform and landform in a single swig. For years I've considered Hertfordshire a shallow landscape, but now I'm learning about its hidden depths. If I'd thought about it earlier, I would have noticed how chalk infiltrates the lives around me, defining the land and its flora and fauna. In creamy-brown nubs that surface in the vegetable beds; in earth that nurtures calcicole species such as deadly nightshade, wild marjoram, field scabious and, of course, the snails; in the aquifer, springs, winterbournes, swallow holes and chalk streams; in the calcium absorbed via my small intestine as I join the cycle of endless reformation. This simple act of drinking binds me to this place physically and emotionally. It no longer seems fanciful to imagine the land is in my bones.

Chalk might be classed as a 'soft rock', but it has its own particular strength. Far from being easily eroded, the chalk hills of southern England have endured for millions of years because of their permeability. Rainfall percolates through the chalk so readily that comparatively little water remains to flow over the surface and consume the landscape. Through its ability to absorb what is thrown at it, chalk prevails. Perhaps I'm not as calcareous in nature as I like to think. But I am learning that strength is not about shunning chronic illness or beating it. For me it has become a question of acceptance and integration. I'm trying to develop the honesty to be myself.

They say when you hit rock bottom, the only way is up. I'd argue when you reach that lowest point, it's worth taking a careful look at the bedrock that broke your fall. Perhaps it might tell you something about where, when, why – even who – you are. The fluidity of life-form-land-form, the promiscuity of the elements that bind us to this world, is wondrous beyond comprehension. It is also tangible and comforting. Part of that timeless dance in which the only certainty is change.

We sit down at the dining room table. Writing-me and anxious-me. We have decided to tackle this together. After many months, we have realised that we need – I need – more help. And finally, I believe I deserve it too. I have visualised this moment many times. Fourteen years after I was first prescribed antidepressants, I look at the innocuous white tablet in the centre of my palm and realise I am not frightened of it anymore. It's just a pill. I wonder if I'll look back in weeks to come and ask myself why I didn't start taking them years earlier. I don't think I will. I am not a patient person, but I have realised these things take their own time.

All it takes is one mouthful of water. Relax. And swallow.

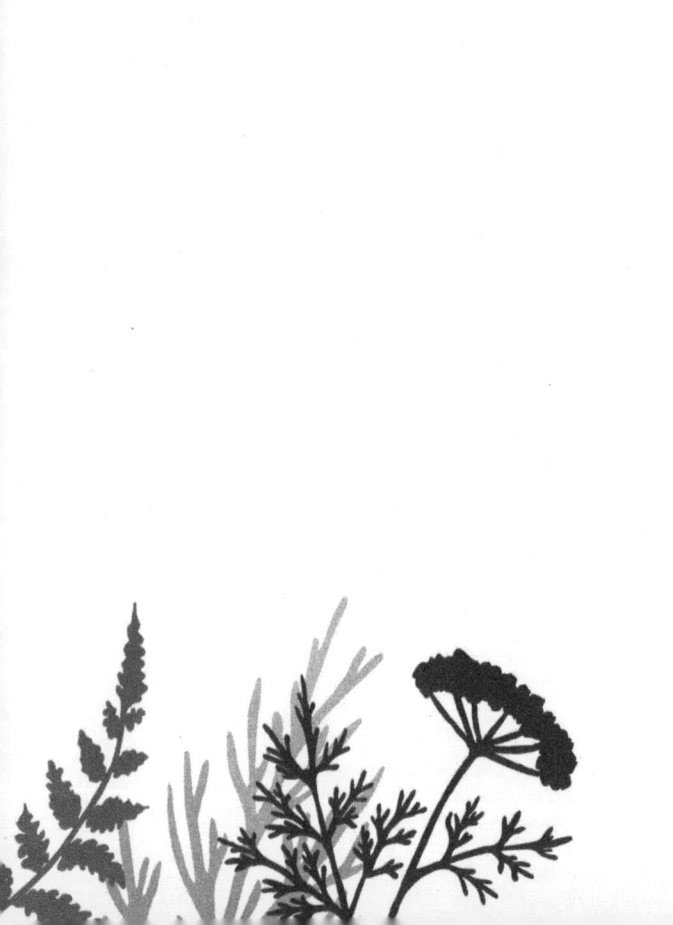

Return to Sea

The Suffolk coast. Six months later.

I'm drinking lukewarm tea in the dark. The sea laps in and out, in and out, rolling sound memories up the beach. I hear soft estuary waves against the hull of my grandpa's boat, while I rock snug and dry in the cabin. Then water slapping the sides of the bathtub and the roar in my ears as my hair is rubbed dry. Further back still and the pulse of life beats through a sphere of saltwater. White noise from an internal world. The sound is comforting, eternal. It steadies me.

I ask the sea for advice.
It answers: Whatever you do, I will keep rolling in and out.
No choice of yours can change me.

Dawn breaks beneath the waves. The yellow light, filtered through grey banks of cloud, reflects off the sea with such intensity it seems to emanate from the depths. In the half-light, yesterday's mark-making is revealed. A montage of footprints in the sand. Different sizes, weights and tread patterns of humans, dogs and birds: diamonds, lines, ellipses; three-pronged gull-prints, too light to see the webbing between the toes; the dainty pawprints of a small dog and the deep-clawed imprints of a far heavier animal. Each step-in-time the record of an individual moment.

Beyond the footprints, a ruined settlement appears. The castle has a dry moat, lowered stone drawbridge and four tubular turrets. It is surrounded by smaller dwellings in various stages of collapse. Soon they will surrender to seawater or trampling feet. Their imminent destruction reminds me that here on the foreshore, reality is fluid. In this littoral kingdom, history exists only between tides, and sound waves submerge you in the past. This plasticity of time reminds me of my doctor's kindly phrase when I told her how desperate I was feeling:

"This moment will pass."

Her compassionate words hung in the air between us. I pocketed them gratefully for later use. She spoke with such conviction. I didn't believe her at the time, but now I know she was right, and I've returned to this particular beach today to fulfil a promise I made a year and a half ago to the sea and myself.

This is the beach where, one windy October morning, Helena and I spotted a small stocky bird foraging on the shingle. In a pebble-dash tumble of rust, tan, brown and grey, white streaks on its wings and a chunky bill with a soft orange shine, it scuttered out from behind a marram tussock. Our first ever snow bunting.

This is the beach where Jamie found a matted lump that looked like something the cat had coughed up. Stranded on the beach after Storm Eunice, we assumed the bedraggled ball was dead but as we watched, it coiled tighter, then slowly unfurled.

It didn't seem a healthy movement, more a slow-motion undrowning. A quick search on my phone gave us a name. Sea mouse. *Aphrodita aculeata.* A species of polychaete or bristle worm sometimes washed up after high tides or storms. Its sandy back had an iridescent rainbow of hairs along the sides that Linnaeus described as 'reflecting the sunbeams from the depths of the sea'. We scooped the spiny goddess of love onto a bed of seaweed and offered it back to the sea, but the waves rolled it up the beach again, so we left the sea mouse in a sheltered rock pool, hoping it would recover, and returned to our sandlarking.

This is the beach where, overwhelmed and rather teary as I grappled with newly evoked memories, a lone sanderling almost ran over my foot. How could I fail to smile through my tears as the little sand-ploughman danced around me, unperturbed by my presence?

This is the beach where the pebbles have eyes, where I borrowed a stone to help anchor me in the present while I excavated the past.

I pull on the hagstone, tugging the necklace out of my shirt and over my plait. Like my tea, it chills quickly in the wind. Numb fingers struggle to untie the leather cord. I slide the stone off the cord and it rests in the centre of my palm. Without its heat, it is no longer a talisman. It is just a pebble. Like all the others around me. It seems ironic that something that has existed for so many millennia and changed so little, except for that central absence, could have tethered me to discrete moments of time, holding mind and body together.

I place the hagstone among the pebbles, some themselves showing the beginnings of holes. The stone I have carried with me all these months settles and blends. When I stand up, it is indivisible from the shingle.

Around half six, the first dog walker passes by. "You scared her," he motions at his dog, "just sitting there not moving." But she trots over for a cuddle anyway, sniffing at my empty tea mug. A second man and his dog are approaching, so I walk up the shingle ridge to leave the beach. On the dunes, sea holly unfurls its softly spiked leaves and freshly emerged sea pea tendrils are on the move. Ahead of me, above the marram grass, I can hear the skylarks singing.

References

Bombweed

'*birds have a Proustian capacity for making remembrance*': John Lewis-Stempel, *Meadowland* (Penguin, 2014), 103.

Moths at Midnight

'*extensive reviews of scientific studies… outcome of the breeding attempt*': BTO Nest Record Scheme Code of Conduct, www.bto. org/our-science/projects/nest-record-scheme/taking-part/coc.

Watcher in the Shadows

'*sang in the trees… in the many quiet pools*'… '*Grendel of old*': Alan Garner, *Weirdstone of Brisingamen* (1960; Collins, 2002), 67, 84.
'*Psallant aethera cum me… Exsultate, Jubilate*': Wolfgang Amadeus Mozart, *Exsultate, Jubilate*, lyrics by unknown author (1773).
'*probably the best musical education available to children between the ages of 9 and 13*': The Choir of King's College Cambridge website, www.kings.cam.ac.uk/choir/choristers.

The Road Less Travelled

'*several times this winter*'… '*much traveled*': letter from Robert Frost to Susan Hayes Ward quoted in *Selected Letters of Robert*

Frost, ed. Lawrence Thompson (Holt, Rinehart and Winston, 1964), 45.

'"Women's Lib forever!"': Robert Westall, *The Wind Eye* (1976; Penguin, 1989), 16.

'A Saint's Life': some of the words in my poem were inspired by Ben Dunwell's libretto for *Saint Cuthbert*, composed by Will Todd, published by Tyalgum Press (1995).

Flatlands

'A cold coming we had... in the very dead of winter': adapted from a 1622 Nativity sermon preached by Lancelot Andrewes, Bishop of Ely and, later, Winchester. It was borrowed (and adapted) by T. S. Eliot as the opening to his poem 'Journey of the Magi' (1927).

'To those who consider... stupendous mountains': Arthur Young, *General View of Agriculture of the County of Hertfordshire* (1804; David & Charles, 1971), 2.

'even tiny amounts... gut damage long term': Coeliac UK website, www.coeliac.org.uk/information-and-support/your-gluten-free-hub/home-of-gluten-free-recipes/new-to-gluten-free-cooking/cross-contamination/.

Grounded

'has been linked... social phobia'... 'loss of the former diet... social activities': C. Rose & R. Howard, 'Living with coeliac disease: a grounded theory study', *Journal of Human Nutrition and Dietetics*, 27 (2014), 30–40 (30). First published in the online journal in 2013.

The Guild of Oca Breeders undertook citizen science trials from 2014 to 2020 to select for early tuberisation and good cropping.

The BFG

'*great joy to many youngsters... bellowed up*': E. Aillie Latchmore, *People, Places and Past Times of Hitchin* (The Author, [c.1974]), 38.

'*bit of Germany... transported to this German colony at Hitchin*': Latchmore, 40.

'*That's not my... tummy is so fluffy.*': reproduced from *That's not my polar bear...* by permission of Usborne Publishing, 83–85 Saffron Hill, London EC1N 8RT, UK. www.usborne.com. Copyright © 2019 Usborne Publishing Limited.

'*king of all the conifers in the world*': John Muir, *The Yosemite* (1912; Sierra Club, 1988), 94.

'*any fool can destroy trees*': John Muir, 'Save the Redwoods', *Sierra Club Bulletin*, 11 (1920), 1–4, https://vault.sierraclub.org/john_muir_exhibit/writings/save_the_redwoods_1920.aspx.

Snickets

An earlier version of part of this chapter was published on the Land Lines Project website and in *Women on Nature*, ed. Katharine Norbury (Unbound, 2021).

'*little narrow strips*'... '*almost the features of a spider's web*'... '*green balks of unploughed turf*'... '*the whole arable area... as its limits would contain*': Frederic Seebohm, *The English Village Community* (Longmans, Green, 1883), 2, 3.

'*... it would take the pen... of our great colourists*'... '*the force with which... of the blow*': Charles W. Quin, 'A Visit to Mr Ransom's Physic Farms', *The Chemist and Druggist*, 4 (1863), 333–338 (334, 336).

'*about a third... field of currant bushes*'... '*Closterium? lunula: circulation... free of chlorophyll*': Joseph Edward Little, unpublished field notebooks in the collection of North Hertfordshire Museum.

'a veritable bacteriologist's soup for the culture of modern germs': Ford Madox Ford, 'Techniques', *Southern Review*, 1 (July 1935), 20–35 (24–5).

'decking and adorning waies and hedges, where people trauel': John Gerard, *The Herball or Generall Historie of Plantes* (Islip, Norton and Whitakers, 1633), 886.

'traveller's joy buds'... 'Much has been written of travel... upon it': Edward Thomas, *The Icknield Way* (Constable, 1913), 129, 1.

'a young tree in the field... symmetrically': Joseph Edward Little, 'Some Hitchin Gardens and Their Trees II', *The Hertfordshire Express*, 9 June 1923.

'upon a line... of the station'... 'the elms fruit[ed]... the production of leaves': Joseph Edward Little, 'Some Hitchin Gardens and Their Trees III', *The Hertfordshire Express*, 4 August 1923.

'it has not the glamour of birch... to write books about': Oliver Rackham, *The Ash Tree* (Little Toller, 2014), 7, extract used by permission of Little Toller Books.

The Nightingale's Tale

'strong in the blade and of a very good colour'... 'an old-fashioned market town... for its nightingales': 'Praying for the Crops', *Cardiff Evening Express*, 16 May 1898, accessed at Welsh Newspapers online.

'Liebe mich... im Dunkeln!' ('Love me, dear heart / Kiss me in the dark'): Brahms, *Liebeslieder Walzer*, lyrics by Georg Friedrich Daumer (1868).

'lost in the mists of time': Valerie Taplin and Audrey Stewart, *Two Minutes to the Station* (Hitchin Historical Society, 2010), 101.

'Wrynecks, Redstarts, Nightingales... these few days': Joseph Ransom, *Naturalist's Notebook*, ed. Val Campion (Hitchin Historical Society, 2004), 28.

All the material from the *Hertfordshire Natural History Society* can be found in the online journals at www.hnhs.org.

All quotations from John Burroughs can be found in 'A Hunt for the Nightingale' in *Fresh Fields* (1884; Houghton, Mifflin, 1896), 77–111.

'high-sounding character'... 'glaring instance'... 'got that name... of the hedge': letter to the *Hertfordshire Mercury and Reformer*, 17 November 1888, accessed in the British Newspaper Archive.

Street Names of Hitchin and Their Origins: Book 1: The Town Centre, ed. Sue Fitzpatrick and Barry West (Hitchin Historical Society, 1997).

'Hitchin claims to be a favourite spot... "nightingale road"': Alfred Kingston, 'Leaves from my Note-book for 1884', *Hardwicke's Science Gossip* (1885), 129–31 (130).

'if, as I am informed... of the old market town': William Percival Westell, *My Life as a Naturalist* (Palmer & Hayward, 1918), 54.

Inundation

'In the wilderness build me a nest... at rest': Felix Mendelssohn, 'O For the Wings of a Dove', lyrics by William Bartholomew, drawn from Psalm 55 (1844).

Chalkbones

'A proper place... compass all around with water': William Ransom, 'An Account of British and Roman Remains Found in the Neighbourhood of Hitchin', *Transactions of the Hertfordshire Natural History Society* (1886), 39–48 (46).

Epilogue: Return to Sea

'reflecting the sunbeams from the depths of the sea': Linnaeus quoted in W. Baird, 'On the Aphroditacean Annelides', *The Journal of the Linnean Society Zoology*, viii (1865), 172–202 (175).

Helpful Websites

Local Wildlife/Environmental Groups
The Wildlife Trusts: www.wildlifetrusts.org
RSPB: www.rspb.org.uk/helping-nature/support-the-rspb/find-a-local-group-near-you
Butterfly Conservation:
www.butterfly-conservation.org/in-your-area
Bat Conservation Trust:
www.bats.org.uk/support-bats/bat-groups
Mammal Society:
www.mammal.org.uk/local-groups/find-a-group
The Conservation Volunteers: www.tcv.org.uk/find-tcv
Friends of the Earth:
www.friendsoftheearth.uk/take-action/join-group-near-you

ME/CFS
The ME Association: www.meassociation.org.uk
Action for ME: www.actionforme.org.uk
ME Research UK: www.meresearch.org.uk

Coeliac Disease
Coeliac UK: www.coeliac.org.uk

Adenomyosis
Endometriosis UK (also covers adenomyosis):
www.endometriosis-uk.org

Functional seizures
Epilepsy Society: www.epilepsysociety.org.uk/about-epilepsy/
what-epilepsy/non-epileptic-functional-dissociative-seizures

Anxiety
Anxiety UK: www.anxietyuk.org.uk
Mind: www.mind.org.uk
NHS: www.nhs.uk/service-search/mental-health/find-an-NHS-
talking-therapies-service
Samaritans: www.samaritans.org

Acknowledgements

With love and thanks to my parents – to Dad, who has spent the last five decades showing me where the wild things are, and to Mum, who taught me that strength comes in many guises. The natural world neither needs nor heeds my thanks, but I'd like to record my immense gratitude for the role it has played in my life, despite its depleted state.

Thanks to Steve Egersdorff for his support and kindness many years ago, and to Cherith Nixon for inspiring me to set out on my literary travels. I'm grateful to Stephen Garner for letting me tell part of his story in mine, and Arwen Gilbert, who helped me remember. Big thanks to Anne Olivant and Linda Fernley, who have believed in me and encouraged me since I was a kid, and to Kathryn Upton, for being someone I know I can always count on.

Michael O'Neill was the best and most broadminded of tutors, and I would love to have been able to show him where his encouragement led me. Dick Watson took us youngsters to the Lake District and gave us the chance to see how landscape and literature interrelate. Thank you for sharing your photographs and memories of a trip we took 30 years ago.

Bridget and David Howlett from the Hitchin Historical Society have answered endless questions, checked my facts and pointed out new avenues of research – thanks to you both and to the society. I'm also grateful to Tim Dye and the Ransom family for their assistance with my research. Mike Toms from the BTO kindly offered advice on the bird ringing section, Martin Ketcher helped with the nightingale chapter, and Ron Austin and Trevor Gunton gave guidance on regional RSPB history from the 1960s and 70s. I'm also grateful to Emma Crawforth, Owen Glyn Smith, Tim Blackburn, Val Campion, Dave Farrow, Rosemary Golding, Monica Hawley, Phil Gates, Stephen Moss, Amanda Susan Rogers, Brian Eversham and Haydon Bailey for their help, and to Sequoia National Forest Ecosystem Staff Officer Gretchen Fitzgerald for her comments and information about the US Forest Service's conservation work.

Thanks to Chris Young, who told me several years ago that I had a book in me, to Helen for helping me revisit my childhood, and to Midge Gillies and Damian Barr for their encouragement along the way. Diane Maybank and Mary Scott – we've been through a lot together and you've helped me develop as a teacher, a writer and a person. Jo Dobson and Sally Goldsmith – what would I have done without you? Thanks for your support, advice and, of course, all the laughter. I'm hugely grateful to Amy-Jane Beer, Kate Bradbury, Simon Kövesi, Katharine Norbury, Louise Kenward, Jon Woolcott and Paul Fleckney, who have given me so much encouragement over the years and helped me believe in myself. And to Sarah Niemann, who was there with the right advice at the right time. Thank you, it made all the difference.

Cheers to my walking mate, Steve Granger, the only person (apart from my dad when he's IDing leaf miners) who walks more slowly than me, especially in fungi season. And the fab Hitchin Nature Network crew – Mel, Dom, Phil, Simon and Chris – for celebrating local wildlife with me and making me chuckle. Huge thanks to my agent, Cathryn Summerhayes, and to Annabel White. And to Debbie Chapman, Rebecca Haydon, Kate Cooper, Jasmin Burkitt, Ross Dickinson, Tess Jolly and Imogen Palmer at Summersdale. It's been a pleasure working with such friendly and caring teams.

Thank you to Nicola Chester for inspiring me to tell my own story in my own voice and for being such a lovely human bean. And heartfelt thanks to Derek Niemann, kindest and most patient of mentors, who is always there when I need him, challenging me to push myself and supporting me with compassion, humour and good advice.

And, finally, to my home team, Col, Jamie and Helena. Ta for everything – for keeping me going, looking after me when I'm struggling and always having faith in me. I couldn't have written this book without you.

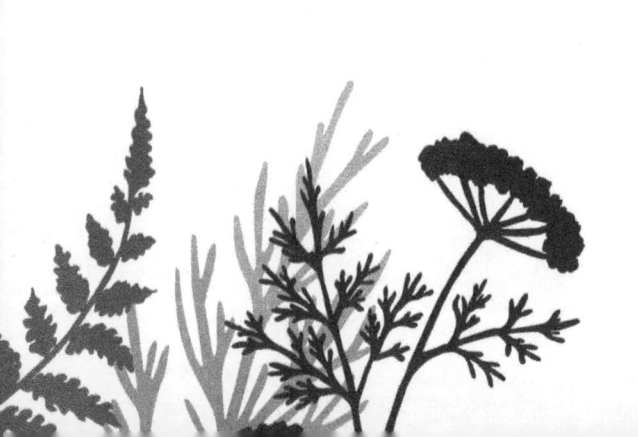

About the Author

Nic has nearly 30 years' writing experience spanning academia, education, journalism and narrative non-fiction. Her qualifications include an MA in English Literature (Open University), a Diploma in Creative Non-Fiction (University of Cambridge) and a Secondary PGCE (Durham University). As well as writing for magazines, websites and anthologies, she also researches the life of Northamptonshire poet, John Clare, and has written the first two of a series of essays on Clare's contemporaries for the *John Clare Society Journal*.

Nic is passionate about connecting people with local wildlife and landscapes. She volunteers for the Herts and Middlesex Wildlife Trust and helps organise a community nature network group. She gives talks and leads workshops on gardening, wildlife and nature writing for a range of organisations including the Wildlife Trusts. She was involved in running the gardening campaign Peat Free April and curated the UK's Peat Free Nurseries List.

When not reading, writing, resting or watching wrens in the reedbeds, Nic enjoys spending time with her family, pottering in the garden, singing in her local choir and making unusual crocheted creatures. Writing *Land Beneath the Waves* has taught her so much, mostly about herself. She tries to be kinder to herself these days and she's learning to pace herself better. Before becoming a writer, Nic spent 12 years teaching English and worked as an A level examiner. She would love to write another book and return to teaching, this time as a nature and life writing tutor.

You can find Nic at www.nicwilson.co.uk, and on Bluesky: nicwilson.bsky.social and Instagram: dogwooddaysgardener.

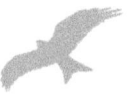

Have you enjoyed this book?
If so, why not write a review on your favourite website?

If you're interested in finding out more about our books,
find us on Facebook at **Summersdale Publishers,** on
Twitter/X at **@Summersdale** and on Instagram and
TikTok at **@summersdalebooks** and get in touch.
We'd love to hear from you!

Thanks very much for buying this Summersdale book.

www.summersdale.com

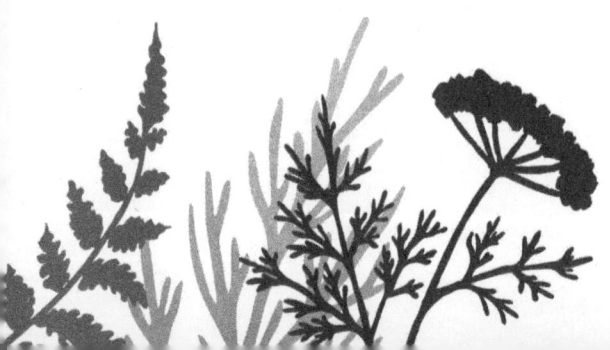